STRUCTURAL INTEGRATION
AND
ENERGY MEDICINE

"In *Structural Integration and Energy Medicine,* Jean Louise Green has created an invaluable tool and guide for those interested in as well as those participating in the process of Structural Integration. Unique in a world of proliferating flavors of body-centered modalities, Structural Integration is at once recognizable as a beacon of hope for those who have run out of options as well as a personal process of self-realization. While it is common for body-centered modalities to focus on clinical symptom relief, Structural Integration goes deeper—focusing on the very core of one's being to deconstruct and then reconstruct the person as an integrated whole. This is a process, and as such, the practitioner serves as both a clinician and guide to the client. *Structural Integration and Energy Medicine* provides both a foundation for understanding the fundamental concepts of the physiologic and scientific aspects of the work and a framework for the conceptual psychological progression that the client experiences over the course of a basic series of the work. This is an invaluable handbook to accompany clients through their ten-session series and provides powerful tools and suggestions to support clients after their Structural Integration series."

MANNY ARAGON, BCSI, PRESIDENT OF THE
INTERNATIONAL ASSOCIATION OF STRUCTURAL INTEGRATORS
AND OWNER OF THE ROLF WORKSHOP

"Jean Louise Green's willingness to share how Structural Integration has affected her and her clients' lives is a beautiful expression of what can happen when your tissues are enlivened. Through her insightful words Green invites you to explore, appreciate, and enjoy the energy field we live in. She shares stories from her practice of many years and gives resources for practical application to embody. Whether you are a Structural Integration practitioner, a Structural Integration client, or a soon-to-be client, this book is a wonderful reference along your journey."

AMBER LEIGH BURNHAM, VICE PRESIDENT OF THE
INTERNATIONAL ASSOCIATION OF STRUCTURAL INTEGRATORS
AND CO-OWNER OF CENTER FOR LENGTH

STRUCTURAL INTEGRATION
AND
ENERGY MEDICINE

A HANDBOOK
OF ADVANCED BODYWORK

Jean Louise Green,
Certified Rolf Practitioner and CMT

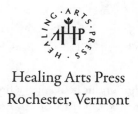

Healing Arts Press
Rochester, Vermont

Healing Arts Press
One Park Street
Rochester, Vermont 05767
www.HealingArtsPress.com

Healing Arts Press is a division of Inner Traditions International

Note to the reader: *This book has been written and published strictly for informational purposes. The remedies, approaches, and techniques described herein are meant to supplement, and should not be a substitute for, professional medical care or treatment or considered to be the practice of medicine. They should not be used to treat a serious ailment without prior consultation with a qualified health-care professional. The author and publisher are providing you with information in this work so that you can have the knowledge and can choose, at your own risk, to act on that knowledge.*

Library of Congress Cataloging-in-Publication Data

Names: Green, Jean Louise, 1955- author.
Title: Structural integration and energy medicine : a handbook of advanced bodywork / Jean Louise Green, Certified Rolf Practitioner and CMT.
Description: Rochester, Vermont : Healing Arts Press, [2019] | Includes bibliographical references and index.
Identifiers: LCCN 2018021856 (print) | LCCN 2018024499 (ebook) | ISBN 9781620557983 (paperback) | ISBN 9781620557990 (ebook)
Subjects: LCSH: Physical therapy. | Mind and body. | BISAC: HEALTH & FITNESS / Alternative Therapies. | BODY, MIND & SPIRIT / Meditation. | HEALTH & FITNESS / Exercise.
Classification: LCC RM700 .G72 2019 (print) | LCC RM700 (ebook) | DDC 615.8/2—dc23
LC record available at https://lccn.loc.gov/2018021856

Printed and bound in the United States by P. A. Hutchison Company

10 9 8 7 6 5 4 3 2 1

Text design and layout by Virginia Scott Bowman
This book was typeset in Garamond Premier Pro, Gill Sans, and Avenir with Tide Sans used as the display typeface.

To send correspondence to the author of this book, mail a first-class letter to the author c/o Inner Traditions • Bear & Company, One Park Street, Rochester, VT 05767, and we will forward the communication, or contact the author directly at **www.JeanLouiseGreen.com**.

◆◆◆

This book is dedicated to Dr. Ida P. Rolf,
Emmett Hutchins, James L. Oschman,
and all teachers and practitioners
of Dr. Rolf's work. May the people of the Earth have the good fortune
to experience the skillful, intelligent, and loving
work of Structural Integration.
May all beings be happy.
May all beings be safe.
May all beings everywhere be free.

Contents

PART I

An Introduction to Structural Integration

List of Illustrations

Acknowledgments

From its inception, the writing of this book had a life of its own. I found myself supported on many levels; the information and help I needed was always there.

With deepest thanks and appreciation, I honor twin sisters Andreini McPherson-Husbands and Andreina Shelton for their artistic contributions to this book. Their insights, cheerleading, and consistent support of this project propelled it all the way from conception to completion. Their generosity of spirit has been essential in the birthing of this project. Thank you for showing up in my life at the perfect time and saying, "YES!"

My partner, Benjamin Hills, brings such joy and beauty to me. He is a foundation of love, support, and care. Thank you for being in my life! And to Ben and all my dear friends, thank you for loving me all these years, even though I had to say "no" many times to keep on track with this project.

With great appreciation, I thank my personal editor, Rosemary Quinn, for her meticulous attention to and passion for the English language. What a lovely dance we had together as we poured over these words! Her work has taken this writing to another level and made it come alive! Carolyn Cameron, thank you for your thorough work on the illustrations and their timely delivery.

Thank you, Randy Peyser of AuthorOneStop, who guided me into the world of publishing and connected me with my perfect publisher. What a blessing you have been for me.

Thanks to Amber Leigh Burnham for her excellent feedback on this manuscript. I also want to acknowledge both Amber and Elisa Jane Noel, current president of the Guild for Structural Integration, for their extraordinary teaching skills and leadership of the next generation of Guild practitioners.

I dearly thank Dr. Ida P. Rolf and all my teachers and mentors of Structural

Integration. I hope this book does justice to the work. Thank you to Emmett Hutchins, Neal Powers, David Davis, Wilhelm Heppe, Stacy Mills, and Sharon Miller. I am grateful for your teachings. Joseph Heller, James Oschman, Robert Schleip, Thomas Myers, Valerie Hunt, Clinton Ober, Betsy Sise, Joe Dispenza, and Richard Podolny—your work has helped me connect many dots.

Thanks to Alan Demmerle for permission to use ten illustrations from *Rolfing: Reestablishing the Natural Alignment and Structural Integration of the Human Body for Vitality and Well-Being* by Dr. Ida P. Rolf. Thanks to Robert Carl Scherzinger, president of the board of directors of Hellerwork International LLC, for permission to use themes and comments along with eight drawings reproduced from the 1990 Hellerwork *Client's Handbook*. Thanks to Book Publishing Company for permission to use the illustration titled Chart No. 3: Composite Picture of the Pattern Forces of the Body and Their Wireless Circuits from the book *Polarity Therapy,* volume 2, by Dr. Randolph Stone. Special thanks to Dr. Richard Podolny, certified by the American Board of Family Medicine and the American Board of Integrative Holistic Medicine and a Rolfing Structural Integration practitioner, for permission to use a section from his poem "Free Balance" in this book.

Special thanks to Dr. James L. Oschman for his encouragement in this project and the writing of the foreword. His work and his insights about the energetics of the human body have been a great inspiration to me.

Thank you to the Structural Integration practitioners who have worked with my body, especially Andrea Dawn Wilson. You have blessed me with your skillful hands and the intentional organizing of my body.

And my clients, each and every one of you—thank you! You have taught me much about compassion and helped me understand the intricacies of myofascial patterning and how to communicate about it.

I also thank my parents, Carl and Rosemary Green, who brought me safely into this world and now carry on their own journeys in the realms of Light. I'd also like to thank my children, Shalin Turner and Mira Lani Heimgartner, for the joy of being a mother and grandmother.

Haidakhan Babaji, my eternal teacher, thank you for guiding the Light within my heart.

Blessings to all!

Foreword

By James L. Oschman, Ph.D.

The concepts presented in this book can benefit anyone and can also enhance the work of all health-care practitioners. The reason for such a bold claim is simple: all healing methodologies and practices affect anatomical balance, whether or not one realizes or intends it. The mechanism? All of the systems in the body are interconnected. Bringing balance to any one system affects all the others. Hence practitioners of Structural Integration/Rolfing need not address pathologies. They align the body vertically, and problems begin to take care of themselves. This is a powerful and effective concept. It works!

This book means a lot to me personally because Structural Integration/Rolfing dramatically changed my life. It gave me a new, unique, and fun profession, along with mental clarity, physical energy, and great health. After experiencing these results myself, I became fascinated with Dr. Ida P. Rolf's revolutionary concepts about reorganizing people's bodies along a vertical line. When I met her in the late 1970s, she challenged me to develop a scientific explanation of her work so that anyone could understand it. I accepted this task and never regretted it.

I did a deep search of the biomedical literature to investigate modern medicine's perspective on Dr. Rolf's ideas about balancing human structure, and I discovered the work of some long-forgotten but very important American physicians from a century ago: Dr. Joel E. Goldthwait and his colleagues at Harvard Medical School, who represent a significant but rarely cited scientific foundation for the modern bodywork and movement therapies developed by Dr. Rolf and others.

Goldthwait, a surgeon, founded the orthopedic clinic at Massachusetts General Hospital, widely regarded as the best hospital in the world. After years of treating patients with chronic problems, Goldthwait concluded that many ailments arise because parts of the body become misaligned with respect to the vertical axis, compromising the function of various organs. The aim of his therapies was to get his patients to sit, stand, and move with their bodies in an appropriate relationship with the vertical axis.

His approach was based in part on observations made while performing surgery on chronically ill patients. He noticed that abdominal nerves and blood vessels were under tension in individuals whose bodies were out of alignment with the vertical axis. He also noted "stretching and kinking" of the cerebral arteries and veins in those whose necks were chronically bent forward. He correlated various cardiac problems with "faulty body mechanics" that distorted the chest cavity in a way that impaired circulatory efficiency. Goldthwait even documented with X-rays the buildup of calcium deposits on the vertebrae of individuals with chronic arthritis and observed that these deposits, often referred to as hypertrophic bone spurs, can diminish when the individual acquires a more vertical stance.

At the time, Goldthwait was reputed to be the best doctor to consult for severe chronic health problems. His therapeutic approach arose from considering the body from a mechanical engineering perspective, in which the proper alignment of parts is essential to reduce wear and stress. In articles published in 1909 and 1911, Goldthwait wrote passionately about how everyone needs to pay more attention to the ways in which they hold and move their bodies in relation to gravity.[1] Goldthwait's ideas were further advanced in studies done by other researchers in 1943 and 1947.[2]

All of this work, however, was done at the dawn of the era of pharmaceutical medicine, and ideas about looking at the body in terms of anatomical balance were soon swept away by the tide of drug-based medicine that continues today.

Structural Integration is a modern approach that offers a way of correcting the causes of our aches and pains by addressing anatomical balance, rather than suppressing symptoms with pain medications. Goldthwait, writing in collaboration with three other physicians from Harvard Medical School in 1934, provides an eloquent and concise biomedical explanation for the successes of Structural Integration:

The way we hold and move our bodies in our daily activities is more important than most people realize. It is desirable to be able to stand erect and to have the parts of the body balanced so that easy and graceful movement occur. These ideas about how we stand and move are important for full health and economic efficiency of the body. The most economical way to use the body is with proper poise. This allows more energy to be available for whatever task is required. Any time a structure departs from the balanced state, energy is wasted and efficiency is reduced. An imbalance can cause one part of the body to be strained more than another, but no one part can be strained without affecting the whole body.

It would seem to be a matter simply of common sense to expect better health with the body so poised or balanced that all of the organs are in their proper positions and the muscles are in proper balance. Likewise with the poise such that the viscera of both the abdomen and thorax must be out of place, as can be easily demonstrated with X-rays, the best health could hardly be expected. The malposition of an organ will disturb its function. If malposition continues long enough, permanent damage will result, but if the faulty mechanics is corrected, damage will be prevented.[3]

Goldthwait's therapeutic process was long and tedious. He would have been enthusiastic about Dr. Rolf's discoveries of the plasticity of connective tissue, which enabled her to accomplish in a few hours what Goldthwait did over a period of many months—for example, by having his patients lie on pillows positioned in ways that gradually coaxed their bodies into better alignment.

The very idea that our living structures can be integrated is fascinating in itself. For athletes, dancers, and other performers, an approach that enables the structural systems in their bodies to work together effortlessly and smoothly—to be integrated—is incredible news. These are individuals whose success depends on developing energy-efficient, easy, and graceful movement. It is no surprise that a number of Olympic medalists and world-champion athletes have acknowledged the importance of Dr. Rolf's work for their accomplishments. But you do not have to be a performer striving for perfection to experience a wide range of benefits from the remarkable process of Structural Integration. Everyone living in the gravity field of our Earth can incorporate these ideas into their daily lives and benefit from them.

For those choosing to experience this path, this book is an excellent preparation for the journey. It is valuable to understand the goals of each session, to know how to prepare yourself for the next one, and to learn how to incorporate the results between sessions. The information Jean Louise Green has organized in this book is priceless.

Green has integrated far more than structure—she has integrated her lifetime of experiences and adventures with human structure, mind, body, and spirit. This is an accurate, concise, and inspired perception of what Ida P. Rolf set out to accomplish.

Having experienced the work and having taken many clients through the process has enabled Jean Louise to have a truly holistic and spiritual perspective, and that is what comes through as you read the book. If you have already experienced Structural Integration, the book will remind you of important outcomes that you may have forgotten or may not have been aware of at the time.

If you are considering having this amazing experience, this book will prepare you like none other. Some of the pieces of this story can be found elsewhere, but this is the place where you will find the whole picture.

James L. Oschman, Ph.D., author of *Energy Medicine: The Scientific Basis* and *Energy Medicine in Therapeutics and Human Performance,* received a bachelor of science in biophysics in 1961 and a Ph.D. in biological science in 1965 from the University of Pittsburgh. In the 1970s Oschman's life changed significantly. Upon meeting Nobel Laureate Albert Szent-Gyorgyi, a fascinating journey began. Having received Structural Integration with Peter Melchior, he was asked by Ida Rolf to assist her in explaining the science behind her work. He accepted and over time became a leading authority in energy medicine, developing the concept of the "living matrix." Nicholas French, a distinguished presenter at the first IASI symposium in 2006, said, "James Oschman makes science alive and accessible."

Preface

Each one of us is an energetic being in a physical body. We are body, mind, emotion, and spirit. As we address one aspect of health, we affect all aspects of health. My teacher, Emmett Hutchins, paraphrased *his* teacher when he stated, "Dr. Rolf said that every psychological problem has a physical counterpart. Working on the physical makes the psyche more easily available. Plasticity of the body goes along with plasticity of the mind." Structural Integration is a form of bodywork created by the pioneering biochemist Dr. Ida P. Rolf, Ph.D., who lived from 1896 to 1979. This practice is also popularly known as "Rolfing," in her honor. It helps to create a more balanced and steady human being and is a springboard that launches a person into their next level of being.

Structural Integration works with the fascial connective tissues of the body. These tissues give the body its shape and surround all the major organs and systems of the body. They are also the pathways for the movement of subtle life force energy; people who are familiar with the organ meridian system of acupuncture know this energy as qi.

Systematically working with the entire body, a practitioner of Structural Integration also works to ensure that connective tissue layers can move freely and smoothly in relation to one another. In doing so, problematic strain patterns can be released to restore proper movement and the structural integrity of the body. To the extent possible, the natural design of the body is restored through a series of ten sessions. Wholeness and integrity emerge, allowing the client to live and express more fully and efficiently. How wonderful it is to release limiting strain patterns and open to new possibilities!

Structural Integration has become a much more gentle process since the late sixties when Dr. Rolf developed it at Esalen Institute in Northern California. As

Certified Advanced Rolfer Betsy Sise put it, "Early on, we Rolfers were not familiar with the paradigm that connective tissue was plastic and could change easily. We believed that you had to work extremely hard for change to happen."[1] Current Structural Integration training about the nervous system, fascia, body structure, and movement informs practitioners how to use a refined quality of touch that brings increasing finesse and precision into their work. Current fascial research, such as that of French hand surgeon Dr. Jean-Claude Guimberteau, is providing new insights into living human connective tissue. We can now see more clearly who we are under our skin. And we do not find the tough, dry, unresponsive tissue of a cadaver. The living matrix of fascia is wondrously beautiful, alive, and ever changing. This understanding of how we view and relate to the connective tissues of the body represents a paradigm shift.

Many of the adaptive, self-organizing and dynamic attributes we may wish to embody are already right there inside us! They permeate our entire being through the liquid crystalline-like matrix of the healthy body-wide fascial web. This understanding of fascia is informing the how and why in the quality of touch and intention of bodyworkers as we assist movement in the tissues and release adhesion in the body.

Structural Integration is *personalized* bodywork that meets each person where they are. According to Dr. Rolf's close associate, Rosemary Feitis, Dr. Rolf "was not interested in curing symptoms; she was after bigger game. She wanted nothing less than to create new, better human beings. The ills would cure themselves; the symptoms would melt as the organisms became balanced."[2]

Stress from the outer world can embed itself in our fascial tissues as patterns of strain. Structural Integration works to release these chronic patterns. As the strain dissipates, pain and inflammation diminish. Related emotional and mental stress may resolve as well. New energy becomes available and increased well-being can emerge.

"I feel really good now!" "I didn't know anything could be done. I'm so happy to be out of pain!" "Finally! *This* is who I am!" These are the exuberant comments of many Structural Integration recipients. These big and little miracles happen every day on Structural Integration tables around the world. For a practitioner, it's all in a good day's work; for the client, it can be life changing.

This handbook is designed for both practitioners and clients of Structural Integration and for anyone who may be interested in learning more about it. For practitioners, this book serves as a useful reference guide for their daily practice, as well as providing insights and explorations into the continuing research and evolution of this technique. For clients, the book serves as an introduction to Structural Integration, an explanation of how and why it works, and a practical handbook for maximizing the benefits of this hands-on approach to healing.

Part I: An Introduction to Structural Integration delves into the basics of Structural Integration, such as how it can correct rotation patterns that contribute to pain and degeneration of joints and discs. Part I also summarizes relevant science regarding the energetics of the Rolf Line.

Part II: The Recipe Sessions goes through each of the ten sessions of Structural Integration in detail. The portions on understanding the Rolf Line, self-care, and movement awareness specific to each session can be used to help you receive and integrate the work more fully, as well as generate better habits to avoid recreating strain patterns.

Part III: Support Tools contains information that can help to minimize putting physical, mental, and emotional stress into the body along with suggestions that can help optimize our human experience.

Dr. Rolf was deeply influenced by her studies of biological science and physics. She recognized the importance of gravity in reinforcing the body's architecture and energy field—particularly if the body is *organized,* as she called proper alignment. "We want to get a man out of the place where gravity is his enemy. We want to get him into the place where gravity reinforces him and is a friend, a nourishing force."[3] To do this, the center of gravity of the major parts of the body need to be symmetrically organized one above the other, around a central vertical axis that Dr. Rolf referred to as the Line.

It is my experience that when the body parts are aligned in Structural Integration and the physical, mental, and emotional stresses are cleared from the connective tissues, access to larger fields of energy open up to us. We are, at heart, energetic beings in a physical body. It is our birthright to be supported, sustained, and nourished by the fields of energy that surround us in every moment of our lives.

Structural Integration holds the potential for vast transformation and evolution if that is what you truly desire. This is the work I am honored to do. I feel that it is the most important gift I could share with anyone.

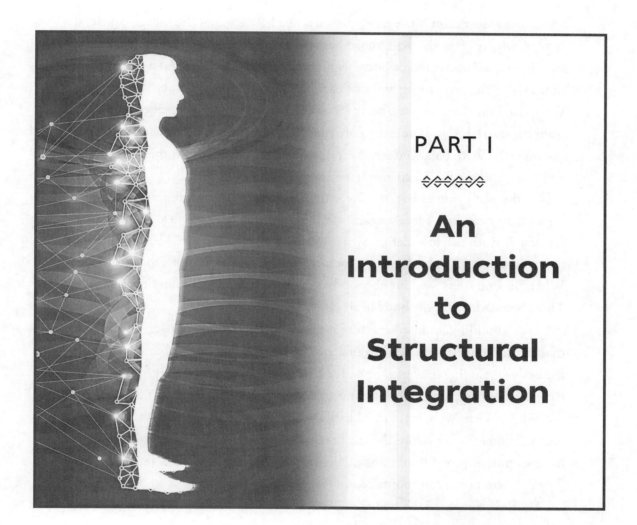

PART I

An
Introduction
to
Structural
Integration

Structural Integration Defined

Structural Integration is the three-dimensional balancing of the musculoskeletal system, which gives rise to a more harmonious relationship with gravity. In a ten-session series, the major body segments are organized around a central vertical axis so the center of gravity of each segment lines up one above the other. Vertical alignment allows the body's muscles to be balanced from side to side and from front to back and for inner core muscles to be balanced with outer superficial muscles. With balanced structure, gravity pulls equally from the front, back, and sides, and the body expends less energy maintaining balance.

As the body moves back to the symmetry of its original design, subtle life-force energy can move freely again, activating the body's own healing processes. Dr. Ida P. Rolf, the founder of Structural Integration, stated, "The unimpeded flow of gravity through a human structure supports and maintains that structure. When the body gets working appropriately, the force of gravity can flow through. Then, spontaneously, the body heals itself."[1]

Like a building, human structure is subject to the laws of physics, which state that masses must be balanced in order to be stable. Eight stackable segments of the body (including the head, neck, torso, hips, upper legs, lower legs, ankles, and feet) are held in place by bones, muscles, and fasciae (connective tissues). Like the World Wide Web, myofascial tissue—that is, the fascia of the muscles (*myo* means "muscle")—envelops the entire musculoskeletal system. Chronically short muscles pull attached bones out of alignment. When the fascia is balanced and repositioned, bones can spontaneously reorient.

Dr. Rolf compared the body's musculature to the structure of a tent, with the pole being the spine.[2] The fabric and lines pulling against the pole from one direction are balanced by the fabric and lines pulling against it in another direction. If the lines are too loose, the tent will sag. If they're too tight, it will torque. With equal tension, the tent will have optimal height and width, and the pole serves simply as a spacer between forces. The lines (muscles) bear the weight of the fabric, not the pole (spine). In the body, this spatial symmetry occurs through proper organization of the fascia.

Fascial tissue is comprised of collagen proteins. It wraps around every muscle and organ, creating various fascial planes and bags that hold the body together. When a fascial structure is injured, it secretes semifluid materials that dry up and become glue-like, which causes tissues to adhere, impeding true movement. When a practitioner of Structural Integration applies energy to the knotted collagen tissues, using their fingers, knuckles, or forearms, the glue seems to dissolve and the muscles release.

"Bodies carry their history written within them," said Dr. Rolf. "In accidents, muscles get displaced slightly, so in continuing to move around, the body uses a different muscular pattern. That different muscular pattern places itself on top of what should be the effective muscular pattern of the uninjured body."[3]

One of my clients, a sports club trainer, gave a classic description of how injuries affect the body:

> People don't understand that it is muscle patterns that are getting them in trouble. They don't understand that the injury they incurred as a fifteen-year-old is lingering and has had a snowball effect. First it's your hip. Then it becomes your foot because your hip is out of alignment; and then the lower back and a shoulder. By the time you know it, there are seven things out of alignment from one issue!
>
> A friend of mine was trying to go the method of lifting weights, jogging, and stretching. Nothing was helping him so I told him, "It's because you are stretching a body that is not aligned!"
>
> Since I have been getting these sessions, my body is becoming aligned and it's allowing me to reach my potential. I don't have any pain! No pain in my hip and I used to have pain to where I couldn't sleep and I would actually hit my hip because it hurt so bad. And now I can bend forward and place my hands on the ground. And I haven't stretched for ten weeks! I just feel amazing.

Structural Integration is a path of personal transformation. With upright posture and structural balance, our confidence naturally builds and our mental state becomes more focused. We are also likely to have more awareness of how we express our feelings and emotions.

"This work helps propel other avenues of your life to become aligned," said a client. "You get mental and emotional benefits as well as physical benefits. It just embodies everything! I remember feeling so calm and in tune with my emotions after some sessions. I was just level-headed and intelligent. It was fun! I could access things because my body wasn't expending energy on pain or thinking about what was wrong. When that is relieved, the body is like, 'Yeah! Finally. Now this is who I am!'"

Dr. Ida P. Rolf, Founder of Structural Integration

Dr. Ida P. Rolf was a pioneering, original mind. She had always investigated what was new and was never afraid to take what she learned and use it.

ROSEMARY FEITIS

Ida Rolf was born in 1896 into the family of a prosperous contractor in the Bronx of New York City. Her father was fully supportive of her strong personality and self-confidence, providing for her higher education and empowering her to succeed in a male-dominated society. She graduated from Barnard College during World War I and obtained a job at the Rockefeller Institute, where she worked for twelve years in the chemotherapy and organic chemistry departments.

In 1916 twenty-year-old Ida Rolf had a life-changing event while camping in the Rockies. She was kicked by a horse, and severe fever and impaired breathing set in. The small-town Montana doctor who initially treated her referred her to a local osteopath. After a simple spinal manipulation, her fever reduced immediately and her breathing became normal.

That simple spinal adjustment demonstrated that freeing obstructions between joints could enhance the body's overall function and well-being. Young Ida Rolf saw that vertical alignment of the head, rib cage, pelvis, and legs affects health, behavior, and consciousness. This incident initiated her study of how structure determines function.[4]

While working at the Rockefeller Institute, Ida Rolf continued her studies and earned a Ph.D. in biochemistry from Columbia University in 1920. This job also allowed her to go to Switzerland, where she studied mathematics and atomic physics in Zurich and homeopathic medicine in Geneva.

During her graduate studies in biochemistry, Dr. Rolf also began to study yoga with a tantric yogi in Nyack, New York. Describing the significance of her studies during this time, which formed the basis of all her future work, Don Hanlon Johnson, Ph.D., says that Dr. Rolf "began to wonder about the connection between the osteopathic notion of vertical skeletal alignment and the ancient notion of the alignment of chakras. She would eventually synthesize certain ideas of Western biology and Eastern spirituality into the notion that access to the furthest reaches of the human potential required removal of the muscular torsions and skeletal imbalances that impede the free flow of various energies such as oxygen, lymph, blood, and neural messages."[5]

With the death of her father in 1928 and a subsequent inheritance, Dr. Rolf began lifelong travels in which she studied various spiritual and physical disciplines. She also taught yoga and applied exercises and manipulative techniques to people in need who came to her.

In 1942 Dr. Rolf started a two-year period of work with a friend, Grace, who had been crippled since childhood. "That day I started working with Grace," said Dr. Rolf, "was the day I really got Rolfing going. That was when the first principle of Rolfing was really born—moving the soft tissue toward the place where it really belongs."[6]

Dr. Rolf developed original ideas regarding manipulation and healing of the human body. She noted that the body is comprised of segmented parts. She also noted that the body can change because of the malleability of its connective tissues. And she realized that the human body has a relationship with the gravitational field.

From 1965 to 1968, Dr. Rolf taught at the Esalen Institute in Northern California. She called her system of work Structural Integration, which she felt described the process of her technique. At Esalen, the nickname "Rolfing" was first coined. In 1967 Dr. Rolf began writing her book, *Rolfing: The Integration of Human Structures*. It was completed in 1977. In 1971 Dr. Rolf founded the Rolf Institute of Structural Integration in Boulder, Colorado.

Dr. Rolf died in 1979 at the age of eighty-three. In describing her accomplishments, Dr. Rolf said with modesty, "One does not get very far in one lifetime." We beg to differ!

As another part of her legacy, Dr. Rolf's work continued to emerge in Boulder, Colorado, with the Guild for Structural Integration, founded in 1989. And in 2002 the International Association of Structural Integrators (IASI) was founded as the professional membership organization for Structural Integration. IASI has recognized many schools of Structural Integration from around the world that are compliant with their current educational standards for Structural Integration. In compliance with IASI standards, a Certification Board for Structural Integration (CBSI) provides a board exam for Structural Integrators.

My Own Journey in Structural Integration

I have been a practitioner of Structural Integration since 1991. I first studied at the Guild for Structural Integration in Boulder, Colorado, with Emmett Hutchins, Stacy Mills, David Davis, and Wilhelm Heppe, and I completed my practitioner training shortly after with Neal Powers in San Francisco, California. Six years later I had the privilege of being mentored by Sharon Miller, one of just thirteen people in the world to be taken through two levels of advanced training with Dr. Rolf. In fact, Dr. Rolf was Sharon's *only* teacher. To my good fortune, Sharon lived close to my office in downtown Hilo, Hawaii, so I had the extraordinary opportunity to work with her regularly from 1997 to 1999, until I moved away.

My introduction to Structural Integration came through other body practices and work. Early training as a gymnast led me to become a gymnastics coach. The desire to be a more effective coach led me to a massage program, where the study of anatomy and kinesiology was the focus for the first six months. During that massage training, I realized that I had a gift with my hands. I also experienced the work of Structural Integration for the first time. After my second session, I looked at my practitioner, David Sigala, and exclaimed, "I am going to do this work someday!" Four years later I was grateful to be in my first training class at the Guild for Structural Integration.

During the core-level work at the Guild in Boulder, my pelvis became horizontal again. I remember that day well, as it was a pivotal moment of great joy and new awareness. When I trained as a young gymnast, my coaches and I were not aware of the necessity of pulling the belly button back toward the spine while doing abdominal conditioning. Not doing so can disorganize the core-level psoas muscles, pulling them away from the spine. This drags the lumbar spine forward and creates an excessive "swayback" curve in the lower back, which the medical community calls *lordosis*. When the lower end of the spine is pulled forward like that, the head and neck usually pull forward as well. This is exactly what had happened to me, and as a result, standing, sitting, and kneeling for periods of time had become uncomfortable. My pelvis was not "at home" in my body.

During that core-level work at the guild, my chronically contracted psoas muscles released. My pelvis dropped, and my lower back lengthened. I felt my body weight drop into my feet for the first time in many years. No longer was it an effort to hold myself up. A sense of ease and relaxation moved through my body. Finally, I was able to let my weight down into the earth so it could support me. What an incredible sense of relief!

After that session I went outside and walked, skipped, and ran with delight. This was what I wanted my body to feel like! The change to a horizontal pelvis was mine to keep and has stayed with me ever since.

After my training, I devoted myself to full-time bodywork. I have spent many hours studying and working with bodies, pondering their anatomy, structure, and function. The ten-session series designed by Dr. Rolf has been the framework of my explorations. My teacher Neal Powers said that it takes about ten years to really know what you are doing. Emmett Hutchins said that being a practitioner of Structural Integration was a spiritual path—a path of purification. I asked him what he meant. He smiled and said, "You'll find out."

I have lived, breathed, and dreamed my craft—and consistently rolled up my sleeves in this work for twenty-five years as a full-time professional. I show up daily at my treatment room, hone my skills, and let the beings on my table teach me. Since 1991, when I was thirty-six years old, studying with master teachers and going through my own personal transformations has been my path.

Being a practitioner of Structural Integration has its own challenges and dilemmas, which Dr. Rolf described as getting secure in an art in which there is no security. As she put it, "A Rolfer's only secure ground in a body is to establish a balanced relationship. That is your secure ground, and it is not possible to convert it into something that is solid like a wall."[7] Dr. Rolf was referring to security in a balanced body and its relationship within the gravitational field.

So in the worldly sense, my craft may seem an insecure one. It is made of the unseeable stuff of energy, principles, and relationships. True security is living within a balanced body that is able to effectively relate to the gravitational field.[8]

I have spent years learning to bring order out of disorganization in the layers of connective tissues in a human body. And yet, I am still passionate about and fascinated by Structural Integration's exploration of the gravitational field as a beneficial force. Dr. Rolf alluded to this possibility, saying:

> Rolfing postulates on the basis of observation that a human is basically an energy field operating in the greater energy of the earth; particularly significant is that energy known as the gravitational field. As such, the individual's smaller field can be enhanced or depleted in accordance with the spatial relations of the two fields....
>
> This is the gospel of Rolfing: when the body gets working appropriately, the force of gravity can flow through. Then, spontaneously, the body heals itself... and gravity becomes the therapist.[9]

During my training in Structural Integration, I learned about the importance of organizing body segments. I understood how gravity could be an unrelenting detrimental force if major body segments were not lined up properly, but the question of how gravity could be an ongoing *beneficial* force eluded me. It seemed that Dr. Rolf was referring to something more than body segments being lined up properly. My mentor, Sharon Miller, seemed to refer to the same phenomenon when she spoke of being able to bring universal energy into the body while we worked so that we could recharge ourselves and feel at home. I had an understanding of those words in my mind, but I still needed an experience I could relate to in my body. Much time has passed since the early days of my first Structural Integration series. I have experienced unusual energy flows in my organized body that I now frame in a new context.

One day in 2007, as I lay in bed reading Betsy Sise's excellent book *The Rolfing Experience,* I came across a couple of paragraphs Sise had reproduced from an unpublished paper in 1989 by her teacher Emmett Hutchins, titled "Structural Integration: A Path of Personal Growth and Development." I felt those words were describing me! They spoke of the free flow of electric core energy through the body when blockages in the physical and energetic levels were removed:

> And what if one were to place the negative pole of this energized core (root chakra) firmly into the earth while also spanning upward through the positive pole (crown chakra) toward infinity?

Would the personal electromagnetic field be reinforced by the field of the earth? Could this not describe a transcendent state of energetic integration between human and cosmos? Could this correspond to awakening of kundalini and the appearance of super-normal powers of mind and body? Are chakras the vortices through which this highly empowered electromagnetic source communicates with matter?[10]

In that moment I had a significant realization. Structural Integration, yoga, meditation, and life experience together had created a new level of connection with Source within me.

In 2006 three hundred Structural Integration practitioners from around the world gathered in Bellevue, Washington, for the first IASI conference. Many different schools of Dr. Rolf's work had evolved over the decades, and it was time to come together to create consistency, set aside differences, and build on our common knowledge. It was a grand reunion for the larger family of Structural Integration.

As Dr. Rolf's close colleague, Rosemary Feitis, ended her opening statement, she asked, "What is gravity?" I don't think she intended for anyone in the large audience to answer her question, but with a pounding heart I found myself raising my hand! Credible or not, I felt compelled to communicate my experiences of my body's relationship with gravity. I hoped my sharing would warrant my colleagues' attention.

As she acknowledged me, I silently prayed, "Oh Lord! Let my words ring clear and true!" As I rose, my feet found strength beneath me. I looked around the entire room and took a breath. A sea of intelligent, thoughtful faces surrounded me. I addressed them all. I began to speak about Earth energy. I spoke of heavenly energy. I described how having a Rolfed body helped me experience the movement of these energy flows: Energy enters through the bottom of my feet and the top of my head. It feels like showers of love that connect me with a sense of home as I link into the greater field of universal energy.

I described how my body would tingle as every cell was bathed in light. I contended that these flows emerge from the electromagnetic field that arises from gravity, and that our bodies can become conscious conduits of the gravitational energy fields.

"When physical, mental, and emotional blockages are removed and the major body segments are aligned, beneficial life force can charge us up. And that's what our work as Rolf practitioners enables us to do for others," I said.

I saw heads nod up and down in agreement. I also saw looks on some faces like, "What the heck is she talking about?" I braved their thoughts and perhaps their judgments. These words needed and wanted to be spoken.

As it was, my words were a perfect segue into the next presentation by James L. Oschman, a biophysicist and the author of *Energy Medicine: The Scientific Basis* and *Energy Medicine in Therapeutics and Human Performance*. He immediately began to describe his ideas on the "living matrix," the ability of our body's connective tissues to transmit and conduct electromagnetic energy at quantum speeds.

I believe it is our birthright to have a human body that can be supported, sustained, and nourished by the fields of energy that surround us—if only we knew how to access them and allow them to flow through us fully! As Dr. Rolf said, "Rolfers make a life study of relating bodies and their fields to the earth and its gravity field, and we so organize the body that the gravity field can reinforce the body's energy field. This is our primary concept."[11]

The Rolf "Recipe"

Over the course of fifty years of observation and experience, Dr. Rolf developed a series of ten sessions of bodywork. She called this series "the recipe" and considered it the culmination of her life's work. Within the recipe is a specific road map for practitioners to balance and remove strain from the layers of connective tissue. Each session has specific goals and intentions. Practitioners customize this recipe according to their client's need.

The recipe has three parts. Sessions 1 to 3 work with the superficial fascia. Session 4 to 7 work with the core-level structures. Sessions 8 to 10 are integrative and customized.

Sessions 1 through 7 are called the *hours of differentiation*. (The word *hour* here means a session.) These sessions work systematically with every part of the body to create more length and space.

Sessions 8, 9, and 10 are called the *hours of integration*. These sessions are customized according to the individual needs of the client. Sessions 8 and 9 address the two girdles—the pelvic and shoulder girdles respectively. Session 10 completes the series by addressing the entire body.

I have found it optimal to work with a person once or twice a week at the most. Spreading the sessions over this time span allows the person's body time to assimilate changes. It also creates the opportunity for the next area of strain to surface. People often notice that they are symptomatic in the areas that are about to be addressed. This is the power of the recipe at work!

Energetics of the Body

The Rolf Line: Conduit of Life-Force Energy

A basic premise of Structural Integration is that the major body segments of the head, shoulders, hips, knees, and ankles are organized around a central vertical axis, or the Line, as Dr. Rolf called it. For a Rolf practitioner, this Line is considered in a *structural* sense because we organize the center of gravity of a person's major body segments around it. Dr. Rolf referred to such segments of the body as "an aggregate of blocks."[12] I also like to think of the Line as being *functional* because it creates an energetic channel for the movement of life-force energy between the electromagnetic fields of the celestial heavens and the terrestrial Earth.

Imagine an energetic Line that begins in the center of the Earth and runs all the way to the heavens. That same Line runs through the center of your feet and legs, up the front side of your spine, through the center of your neck, and out the top of your head as it continues into the heavens. Through that Line, the body becomes a conduit for larger fields of energy. Breath activates this Line.

The Taoists of ancient China studied universal life-force energy, also known as *qi* (pronounced "chee"). The word *qi* means energy, air or breath, vitality, or universal force of life. The Taoists said that there are two main sources of energy on our planet: heavenly energy and earthly energies. Our bodies are surrounded and penetrated by these energies. We become aware of them when we experience our Line. The force of these energies is electromagnetic and arises out of the gravitational fields in which we live. They help nourish, support, and maintain our physiological systems. In this way, like a living crystal, the human body can be charged and renewed.

We call this type of awareness "being on our Line." Via the Line, we can experience energetic renewal and personal empowerment through conscious connection with the larger energy fields of the heavens and Earth.

On a subatomic level, electromagnetic energy flows around the body in a doughnut-like shape known as a *torus*. In the center of the torus is the *pranic tube,* a column extending from the crown of the head down through the center of the body to the perineum, which is midway between the anus and the genitals. It is an energy channel for connecting celestial and terrestrial energies. The channel follows the central axis of the body's magnetic field and is approximately the size of the circle formed when you put your thumb and first finger together. The pranic tube is synonymous with the Rolf Line.

From the pranic tube, electromagnetic energy is channeled into energy centers along the spine known as *chakras.* At the chakras, the energy is spun out into the major organs of the endocrine system that produce hormones and then into the meridian system. The meridian system lies within the fascial planes of the body's connective tissues and consists of electrical circuits or pathways that carry this subtle energy throughout the body. As that energy radiates out from the body into a person's energy field, it forms the aura.

Randolph Stone, the founder of Polarity Therapy and another pioneer in the relationship between structure and energy, described the pranic tube as the "ultrasonic core" (see fig. 1.1). He says, "The fine white line in the central core is the ultrasonic energy current of the soul. It is the primary energy which builds and sustains all other."[13]

The Emerging Science of Connective Tissue

Only a thin line lies between science and metaphysics. In this regard, Dr. Rolf once said, "All this metaphysics is fine, but be mighty sure you've got physics under the metaphysics."[14]

Practitioners of traditional Chinese medicine have talked about qi and its movement through the body via the meridians for centuries. Modern science supports the idea that the body is suffused with currents of electromagnetic energy. But what are the mechanisms driving the movement of this subtle life-force energy or qi as it moves through the body?

Biophysicist James Oschman has studied connective tissue and the movement of life-force energy through the body.* Through his studies of biochemistry and

---

*In this section, the words "connective tissue" refer primarily to the connective tissue in general, including fascia, tendons, ligaments, cartilage, adipose tissue, and even bones.

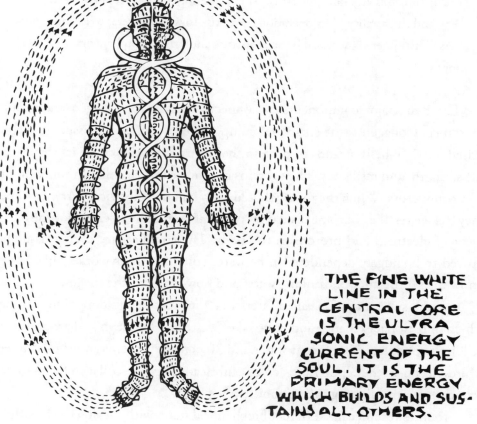

COMPOSITE PICTURE OF THE PATTERN FORCES
OF THE BODY AND THEIR WIRELESS CIRCUITS.

ULTRA-SONIC
CORE

THE FINE WHITE
LINE IN THE
CENTRAL CORE
IS THE ULTRA
SONIC ENERGY
CURRENT OF THE
SOUL. IT IS THE
PRIMARY ENERGY
WHICH BUILDS AND SUS-
TAINS ALL OTHERS.

♦ Fig. 1.1. Image of Randolph Stone's "ultrasonic core."
From *Polarity Therapy: The Complete Collected Works on this Revolutionary Healing Art by
the Originator of the System*, volume 2, by Dr. Randolph Stone, D.C., D.O. (Summertown,
Tenn.: Book Publishing Company, 1987).

the energetics of complementary healing practices, Oschman has developed a
hypothesis about how the connective tissues of the body conduct subtle life-force
energy in what he describes as the "living matrix."

It looks to me, from my study of biophysics and cell biology, like the body is
designed with a semi-conductive fabric that connects everything in the body,
including inside of every cell. I refer to this system as the living matrix. All forms

of energy are rapidly generated, conducted, interpreted, and converted from one to another in sophisticated ways within the living matrix. It delivers energy and information at the fastest possible means that nature has available. No part of the organism is separate from this matrix. Memories are stored within this system, and the totality of its operations gives rise to what we refer to as consciousness. This system is accessed by acupuncture and other complementary medical approaches.[15]

The two major components of connective tissue are collagen and ground substance. Collagen is the structural component of connective tissue. It is comprised of triple-helix strands of protein that give connective tissue its shape, tensile strength, and resiliency. The proteins that make up the collagen function like semiconductors: When they are hydrated, they conduct electrical currents. When they lack water, they become insulators. Water is absolutely essential for the movement of electrons and protons in the body. The conductivity of any tissue has proved to be hugely dependent on its water content.[16] Bodyworkers like myself know the significance of drinking water and how it affects the tissues.

Ground substance, also called interstitial fluid, is the liquid medium through which nutritional exchange and removal of waste takes place in and around every cell in the body. It is 70 percent water and 30 percent proteins and similar to egg whites in consistency. This fluid acts as a lubricant between collagen fibers to prevent them from adhering to one another.

Ground substance has different biochemical states with varying levels of fluidity. Oschman suggests that ground substance forms a continuous supramolecular network extending throughout the body into every nook and cranny.[17]

Oschman's work draws from a new collaborative science based on geophysics, biophysics, electrical engineering, electrophysiology, and medicine that has emerged since Dr. Rolf's passing in 1979. She would be pleased to see that it validates her theories about the gravitational field and its support of the human body.

Electrical Currents and Magnetic Fields of the Body

Since connective tissue plays a part in the movement of life-force energy through the body, let's look at the electrical fields from which those life-force energies arise.

Valerie Hunt, author of *Infinite Mind* and a physicist and physiologist known for her pioneering research on the human energy field, stated, "Although we cannot explain life, we do know that electrical activity is essential to life. All cells, even subatomic particles, contain electrical elements. When the tiny mass of an electron spins around the nucleus of an atom, a magnetic field is created by its spin."[18]

On December 6, 2008, I had the rare opportunity to attend a lecture at the Dominican University of California in San Rafael by Dr. Horst Michaelis, then director of the Academy of BioEnergetics in Liechtenstein. At that time, Dr. Michaelis had been exploring the therapeutic use of pulsating electromagnetic fields for eighteen years. He described how the body is a biomagnetic organism that produces and uses electromagnetic impulses to regulate cell and tissue growth. He said, "Every living being has electrical currents running through it that regulate the body's life processes. Those electrical signals govern the functioning of that body."

In other words, the cells in our bodies communicate through the language of electrically charged impulses. Our physiology relies on the transfer of those electrical charges, or currents. Electrical currents are produced within the body by the activities of the heart, brain, muscles, and other organs.

In his book *Energy Medicine in Therapeutics and Human Performance,* James Oschman refers to two basic laws of physics that demystify electricity and magnetism and their role in the human body. The first of these is Ampère's law. Between 1820 and 1825, French physicist, natural philosopher, and mathematician André-Marie Ampère quantified a fundamental law of electromagnetism: "Ampere's Law states and *requires* that electrical currents such as those produced within the body by the activities of the heart, brain, muscles, and other organs, *must* produce magnetic fields in the space around the body."[19]

Of all the organs, the heart generates the most electricity in the body, with each beat sending 2.5 watts of electricity out into the body by way of the salty blood and extracellular fluid, both of which are good conductors of electricity. Because electrical current *must* produce a magnetic field, the heart also emanates the strongest electromagnetic field in the body. Dr. Karl Maret, a practitioner of integrative medicine who also holds a master's degree in electrical engineering, describes the heart as the "synchronizing electromagnet master clock" around which our bodies organize.[20]

Electromagnetic energy moves through the body. We cannot see it, but it is there. Biomagnetism, the study of the magnetic fields produced by tissues and organs, and magnetobiology, the study of the effects of magnetic fields on living things, use technologies that now enable us to measure these biological electromagnetic energy fields in the body. The magnetocardiogram, for example, measures the magnetic field of the body and generally detects this field extending to a distance of 12 to 15 feet away from the body. The electrical field of the heart, measured by the electrocardiogram, can be picked up on the surface of the skin. The electroencephalogram measures the much smaller electrical fields produced by the brain.

The second basic law of physics that Oschman highlights is called Faraday's law of induction. It's named for English scientist Michael Faraday, who in 1831 demonstrated that "moving or time-varying magnetic fields in the space around the body must induce current flows within the tissues."[21] In other words, not only does an electrical current generate a magnetic field (Ampère's law), but movement or variation of a magnetic field will produce an electrical current (Faraday's law).

Faraday's law is significant in that it proves that magnetic devices can stimulate the body's electrical fields and thus physiological processes. The same principle underlies the practice of healing touch: Medical research has shown that the biomagnetic fields generated by the heart of a practitioner can actually flow through their fingertips and stimulate a subtle electrical response in the tissues of the client.*

The Body as an Energy Field

Valerie Hunt, a research scientist best known for her pioneering work in the field of bioenergy, noted, "Each material substance, living or inert, mineral or chemical, has its own vibratory signature. These particles form organized patterns of electro-magnetic energy known as a field. Einstein's Unified Field Theory states that all matter is organized energy, and that if all matter disintegrated, we would be left with a field, the primary source."[22]

In fact, a number of distinguished scientists have suggested that what we refer to as matter is actually a local condensation of energy. In this regard, Einstein stated, "We may therefore regard matter as being constituted by the regions of space to which the field is extremely intense. . . . There is no place in

---

*Research on this can be found at the HeartMath Institute, www.heartmath.org.

this new kind of physics both for the field and matter, for the field is the only reality."[23]

According to Hunt, the human energy field is active and reactive. "Although composed of the same electrons as inert substance," she says, "the human field absorbs and throws off energy dynamically. It interacts with and influences matter, whereas fields associated with inert matter react passively."[24]

That energetic interaction with our environment is a natural human characteristic, according to Hunt: "The healthy body is a flowing interactive electro-dynamic energy field. . . . A field is a flowing thing. It flows within itself, through it to other fields, and as an organized unit, it also flows from one place to another."[25]

What's interesting is that human energy fields will respond to an electromagnetic field before our brain and nervous system are even aware of it. The moment we walk into a room, our energy field affects the energy field of everyone else in the room, and vice versa. The flow of electrical current between us is a natural physiological response. This means that healing—the reinforcement of electrical flow in a person—has the potential to happen before a healer has even touched a client.

As Hunt put it, "The reality of the world lies in fields which interact with other fields of energy in dynamic chaos patterns that are always evolving to higher levels of complexity."[26]

The Electromagnetic Field of the Earth

Like the human body, the Earth has an electromagnetic field that flows around the planet in the doughnut-like shape of a torus. This field arises primarily as a result of the flow of molten metals (including iron and nickel) at the Earth's core. The movement of these liquid metals generates electrical currents, and as we've discussed, electrical currents generate magnetic fields.

The force of a magnetic field is measured in units known as tesla. Research shows that a field must have a force of 30 to 200 microtesla to cause a measurable physiological effect on the body. The electromagnetic field of the Earth falls well within that range. The Earth's strongest electromagnetic fields register approximately 66 microtesla at both the north and south magnetic poles. This force decreases with distance away from the poles. It is weakest at the equator, where it is 26 microtesla and farthest from both poles.

The Torus: Breath of the Universe

In 1918, German physicist Max Planck received the Nobel Prize for his discovery that the universe releases light and electromagnetic waves as little packets of wholeness, which Planck called "quanta" ("quantum" for singular).*

The energy of the quanta moves in a specific pattern that mathematicians call the pattern of the torus. The shape of the torus is a three-dimensional doughnut-like shape with a central column down the middle.

In the film *Thrive: What on Earth Will It Take?* the energy of a torus is described: "Energy flows in through one end, circulates around the center, and exits out the other side." In the same film, Duane Elgin, a futurist and author of *The Living Universe,* described how the universe is rolling out these self-organizing torus systems at every scale. "The universe is a torus growing factory," said Elgin. This pattern can be seen in the structure of an atom, in the cross section of an orange, in the magnetic field around the human body or the Earth, and so on, all the way to the galactic level in the shape of spinning galaxies.

---

*For more on Max Plank visit "Important Scientists" on The Physics of the Universe at www.physicsoftheuniverse.com/scientists_planck.html.

Hunt referred to the light and electromagnetic waves that Planck discovered when she spoke about how this energy enters the body. She stated, "[E]xternal electromagnetic energy penetrates the body through acupuncture points and flows through the meridians into the whole field."[27] Our bodies are continually in the presence of this life-enhancing energy of gravity. By consciously drawing the electromagnetic energy into our bodies through our Line, the systems of our bodies are enhanced.

As the energy enters, the piezoelectric property of our semiconductive connective tissues moves this gravitational life force through our bodies. Piezoelectricity refers to "pressure" electricity because every movement, pressure, and tension anywhere in the body "generates a variety of oscillating bioelectric signals or microcurrents through the tissues . . . into cells" of the living matrix.[28]

Oschman surmises that "All forms of energy are rapidly generated, conducted, interpreted, and converted from one form to another in sophisticated ways within the living matrix."[29]

Connective tissue seems "to dictate the flow of electromagnetic energy through-out the body at the finest level," said Hunt.[30] She goes on to say, "Apparently, for all systems to be 'go,' a rich electromagnetic field must be present."[31]

The Earth, too, has a rich electromagnetic field. Scientists have determined that on a subatomic level, the surface of the Earth is covered with a vast reservoir of energy created by the movement of tiny subatomic particles or waves of free electrons that have a negative charge—that is, electrical currents.

Clinical studies show that the physiology of the body synchronizes and responds to the various frequencies in this energy field.[32]

In the foreword of the book *Earthing*, James Oschman explained that walking, sitting, or standing barefoot on the ground for a half an hour or so will activate an electrical exchange between the Earth and our bodies that will restore and maintain the human body's most natural electrical state by optimizing our physiological functions and the health of our bodies.[33] He said, "The Earth is like one gigantic anti-inflammatory, sleep booster, and energizer all wrapped up in one."[34] When connecting with the Earth energy, you'll feel a subtle tingling sensation or warmth rise up your feet. The free electrons of the planet's electrical currents enter the body through the bottom of bare feet and are distributed body-wide through the liquid ground substance of the connective tissues. Their negative charge will neutralize the positive charge of free radicals. This wipes out the inflammation created by free radicals.

Ober stated, "The negatively charged free electrons restore the body's natural internal electrical stability and rhythms, which in turn promotes normal functioning of body systems, including the cardio-vascular, respiratory, digestive, and immune systems. It remedies electron deficiency to reduce inflammation—the common cause of disease. It shifts the nervous system from a stress dominated mode to one of calmness and you sleep better."[35]

The Interstitium and Fascial Research

In May of 2018, a client excitedly swooshed into my treatment room exclaiming, "Jean Louise! I just read some big news on the internet about a new body organ scientists have discovered that they're calling the interstitium. I think it is the same thing as the fascia you've been talking about!" The interstitium buzz had begun, and it followed me later that month to Salt Lake City, where the training I was participating in included a cadaver lab.

The article my young client was referring to, "Structure and Distribution of an Unrecognized Interstitium in Human Tissues," was published online March 27, 2018, in the journal *Scientific Reports*.[36] Around the same time Sarah Gibbens, a digital writer at National Geographic, wrote in her article "New Human 'Organ' Was Hiding in Plain Sight," that researchers from New York University's School of Medicine described the interstitium as "like a mesh. The interstitium is a layer of fluid-filled compartments strung together in a web of collagen and flexible protein called elastin."[37] Some scientists had previously missed this connective tissue because they had been studying dead, dehydrated tissue samples where the fluid-filled compartments had collapsed and flattened, making them difficult to see.

At the time these articles were written, information on the interstitium, or fascia as it is also called, was news to much of the general public. However, this was not a surprise to the experienced hands-on manual therapists, the scientists that had been studying connective tissue for years, or the Fascia Research Congress.*

Thomas Myers, author of *Anatomy Trains* and coauthor of *Fascial Release for Structural Balance*, describes fascia in this manner: "all the bluish-white fibrous tissue that surrounds the muscles, joints, organs, and neurovascular bundles—are all manufactured and extruded into the intercellular spaces by the fibroblasts (fiber-making cells) and their cousins (including osteoblasts, chondrocytes, and mast cells). This comes close to describing what most people understand as the fascial system."[38] Connective tissue has both structural and fluid components. The collagen protein fibers are the structural component of connective tissue. They lie within a fluid gel-like matrix also referred to as ground substance. Myers described this fluid component when he stated, "But then we have to add in all the gels or glycosaminoglycans (GAGs). . . . These hydrophilic sticky viscous gels are a very adaptable part of the fascial system and critical to understanding its properties in training and rehabilitation."[39]

In 2007, participants at the first Fascial Research Congress in Boston defined fascia as "all collagenous, fibrous connective tissue that can be seen as elements of a body-wide tensional force transmission network."[40]

---

*For more information on past and future Fascial Research Congresses, visit www.fasciacongress.org.

Long before all of this, Dr. Rolf played a major role in the awareness of fascia or connective tissue. In addition to the proliferation of training institutes devoted specifically to Structural Integration, Dr. Rolf's concepts and methods now influence a far wider range of other contemporary manual therapies. A growing number of organizations at the local, national, and international levels offer training in "Structural Massage" or in techniques of fascial manipulation that are clearly derivative but focus on the treatment of specific symptoms. Such techniques are increasingly being used by massage therapists, chiropractors, and physical therapists, thus popularizing techniques developed by Dr. Rolf.

Jean-Claude Guimberteau

The debut of Jean-Claude Guimberteau, MD, and Colin Armstrong's book, *Architecture of Human Living Fascia* in 2015 astounded many in the worldwide fascial community. Guimberteau, a French hand surgeon, filmed human living connective tissue with a high-resolution video fiber-optic endoscope. His work brought forth images of human living fascia that were radically different from those normally seen in books and cadaver studies.

With his patients' consent, Dr. Guimberteau used a tourniquet to stop blood flow for fifteen to twenty minutes during surgeries he was performing. The endoscope with its tiny camera was then inserted to take a look around between the tissues. What he found astonished even him!

Beautiful fluid-filled interstitial spaces that he termed microvacuoles and chaotic fractal patterns of continuous fibers met his eyes. "One gradually realizes that the body is shaped by a fibrillar network at every level, from macroscopic to microscopic, and from superficial to deep," he reflected.[41]

"Beneath the skin," said Guimberteau, "there are many defined anatomical structures, but between them, the connective tissue has no conceivable order. Instead, there is a completely disorganized network of collagen fibers with a diversity of shapes and a combination of fractal and chaotic patterns."[42]

In response to a pressure or force from outside the body, the fibers would slide and "move independently in different directions and at different speeds while maintaining the stability of the tissue."[43] They appeared to be dispersing and spreading out vectors of force and energy through the fascial network. What seemed like chaotic movement of fibers and fluid-filled spaces was actually an orderly transmission of strain. Guimberteau proposed that "our bodies function as one dynamic tissue continuum," and he said that fascia could be considered as the "fractionalized tensional architectural network of the human body."[44]

Szent-Gyorgyi and Proteins as Semiconductors

Nobel Laureate Albert Szent-Gyorgyi was one of the leading scientists of the twentieth century who fled his homeland in Hungary in 1947. In 1972 he became James Oschman's mentor after they met at a lecture Szent-Gyorgyi was giving in Woods Hole, Massachusetts. His research was unprecedented, and his remarkable ideas were sometimes met with skepticism. Modern research has since verified the accuracy of many of Szent-Gyorgyi's insights on what is now recognized as the interstitium.[45]

In his keen study of the natural world, Szent-Gyorgyi suspected that there must be another mechanism of response in the body that was much faster than that of the slow movement of bulky molecules. An awareness of quantum physics began entering into his biological focus.

Biochemistry experiments at that time were studying centrifuged, dehydrated proteins. Scientists were more focused on the water-soluble molecules in the upper part of the test tube. Szent-Gyorgyi began studying the stuff at the bottom of the test tube that most scientists were throwing away. These were the proteins of the connective tissues of the body. Albert Szent-Gyorgyi described these proteins as "the stage on which the drama of life is enacted."[46]

Szent-Gyorgyi saw that the proteins of the body had *liquid crystalline-like formations* and surmised that when hydrated, they could become semiconductors of very small, fast-moving particles such as electrons and protons. Electrons conduct the flow of electricity in the body. Protons conduct the flow of energy generated by the mitochondria, the powerhouse of the cells.[47] Other scientists had been missing the hydration factor. Or as Oschman put it, "Take water away, and you are studying nonlife. Keep the proteins hydrated, and they are semiconductors."[48]

In 1968 Szent-Gyorgyi came out with his book *Bioelectronics* where he suggested that the proteins of the body are semiconductors. Here was the joining of biology and physics that provided a rationale for his natural observations. Other scientists at the time also verified such findings.

Oschman took Szent-Gyorgyi's ideas a step further when he stated, "There must be a high-speed communication system in living systems that is *not* the nervous system; instead it is a body-wide energetic communication system that includes the nervous, circulatory, and immune system, and it also includes *all* of the other systems in the body. This *system of systems* has come to be called the *living* matrix."[49]

Mae Wan Ho and her colleagues in Britain also did brilliant work on the liquid crystalline properties of connective tissue. Oschman referenced a study done by Ho in 1993, noting, "It is not generally appreciated that virtually all of the body structure is composed of liquid crystals capable of sustaining quantum coherence."[50] Oschman further quoted Ho directly from her 1999 study, where she stated, "Liquid crystallinity gives organisms their characteristic flexibility, exquisite sensitivity and responsiveness, thus optimizing the rapid, noiseless inter-communication that enables the organism to function as a coherent, coordinated whole."[51]

Water Is the Key

Another key scientific researcher of fascia is the director of research of the European Rolfing Association, Robert Schleip, Ph.D. He began his fascial journey as a hands-on practitioner of Structural Integration and then decided to become an academic scientist to study fascia in the laboratory.

I had the privilege of meeting Schleip at a "Fascial Fascinations" seminar in 2006 in Plano, Texas, where he presented his laboratory findings, which have informed practitioners and clients about the significance of fascia and water. During the seminar, Schleip said that under the microscope, fascia looks like cables of collagen in a gel matrix that is half liquid and half crystalline.

Schleip stated that 67 to 68 percent of fascia is water. He said that the mineral content of the water in the fascia is closer to that of the original oceans. "We have preserved primordial ocean in our bodies," said Schleip. To build up the water content in the connective tissue, Schleip emphasized the importance of the body having a healthy electrolyte content.

He also said that fascia can regulate its hydration. It can swell with water, and it can dry out. Schleip compared fascia to a sponge and said that when you squeeze it out, it fills up again and becomes much fuller in its water content. That's why manual therapy helps the tissue "fluff up." This explains the sensations reported by clients on the treatment table when they describe areas of their body that have been addressed as feeling "fuller" or "more expanded."

"The connective tissue matrix is the interface between our metaphysics and physiology," said Schleip. I was pleased that he encouraged practitioners to channel the expansive good energies of gratitude, love, and appreciation into the connective tissues of our clients as we do our work.

All of this work leads to the understanding that manual therapies that release strain in the connective tissue and help organize the fibers may support a very strong biomagnetic field in the body.

Many thanks to the work of Guimberteau, Szent-Gyorgyi, Oschman, and Schleip, who have helped me connect the dots in order to understand the movement of life-force energy in my own body. I can now strongly affirm that with adequate minerals, proper hydration, and organization of the living matrix of the connective tissue, the electromagnetic field of my body is enhanced and the energies of gravity have become a beneficial force!

Fascial Tissue and Rotation Patterns

In Structural Integration, "The main thing we are after is length and extension: balanced extension," said Emmett Hutchins. "Every movement should be an extension in space. Our enemy in the body is that we get short. We protect ourselves. We get small. There is only one way to get small: Rotation!" So if something is shortening, rotation is involved.

Patterns in the body do have a way of perpetuating themselves. Rotation patterns particularly need to be understood, recognized and addressed. They are so prevalent and yet often unidentified or misunderstood. Painful conditions in tissues and joints may be preceded by connective tissue that have shortened, compressed, and dehydrated because of rotation. Such rotation patterns can lead to degeneration in tissues and joints and may play a significant role in the current epidemic of knee and hip replacements in America. They may also contribute to the prevalence of degenerative spine disorders in aging populations—as the supportive fascia deteriorates, the vertebral discs deteriorate as well.

Barry Nutter, a chiropractor and Structural Integration practitioner, attended a training in Kauai that I participated in. He said that he noticed through X-rays that "if you look at degeneration of the spine over time to see how people age and the discs thin, the problem itself is because of the fascia.

The fascia around the disc deteriorates and loses its circulation and then the bone deteriorates."

Healthy connective tissue supports the structures embedded within it by delivering blood flow, nutrients, neural impulses, and energetic messages and by removing metabolic wastes. When connective tissues become twisted in rotation, they can shorten, compress, and dry out. This dehydration leads to a buildup of metabolic wastes that cause inflammation, pain, and degeneration. The fascia can also adhere to itself or other structures, distorting the shape of the three-dimensional fascial web of the body. This pulls body segments and bony structures out of alignment.

Fortunately, the same pliability of the connective tissue that allows rotation patterns to set in also allows practitioners to skillfully use their hands to loosen fascial adhesions through controlled direction and pressure of movement in the tissues.

Rotation in the body can be present at a micro level or extend into the macro level. It can involve bundles of protein strands in a single muscle group, one or two joints, or whole limbs and girdles of the body. Rotation most often arises from patterns of strain due to injury, poor posture, or repetitive movements.

A rotational pattern of strain affects the body from side to side and from front to back. Its effects tend to manifest in the joints. As my teacher Neal Powers told me, "The joints take up discrepancies in width and length." For example, a rotation can begin in the core of the body with a lifting/twisting injury that affects the spine. It could also begin with a simple ankle twist. Such a twist can pull upward through the fascial planes and joints of the body in a domino effect, creating twist in the knee, pelvis, or spine above it.

Rotations in the body at whatever level are bad news! But they often can be effectively resolved with intelligent, thorough bodywork. And while it is essential for bodywork practitioners to know how to address rotations, it is also important for clients to understand how rotation patterns may contribute to their pain. Then they may be able to minimize activities that perpetuate such twists in their body. For example, if a person has a rotation pattern that goes from right to left, the right leg would be internally rotating and the left would be externally rotating. With such a twist, this person may not want to sleep on his or her left side because that is the direction of the rotation pattern. Sleeping on the right side might be a better choice, as that would help neutralize the twist in his or her body.

Dr. Rolf believed that keeping the fascial planes open is basic to good health because all the major systems of the body are embedded within the connective tissues. Rolf stated, "Fascia is the organ of posture.... [W]e as Rolfers must understand both the anatomy and physiology, but especially the anatomy of fascia. The body is a web of fascia. A spider web is in a plane; this web is a sphere. We can trace the lines of that web to get an understanding of how what we see in a body works. For example, why when we work with the superficial fascia, does this change the tone of the fascia as a whole?"[52]

Dr. Rolf emphasized the importance of paying attention to the joints and mesodermal tissue of the body when she stated, "It's the fascia that crosses joints, not the muscles. Fascial envelopes cross joints. *Joints become the red flag;* they tell you if and how something is wrong. You have to look for relationships, not only of joints, but within all the mesodermal tissue."[53] Mesodermal tissue includes bone, cartilage, fascia, and muscle. They arise from the middle embryonic layer of an animal during its early development.

Connective tissue is patterned by forces of stress and injured in the strains and sprains of muscles, tendons, and ligaments. If it doesn't bounce back with a good night's sleep after a normal day of wear and tear, it needs to be addressed. Skilled hands can assist in restoring balance in an area of fascial strain.

Connective Tissue: Types and Functions

+ Connective tissue, also known as fascia, is the web-like tissue that pervades the body, giving it form and shape. It is continuous in the body, connecting from scalp to sole and from skin to marrow.

+ There are three major layers of connective tissue within the body: the superficial fascia, the deep fascia, and the subserous fascia.

1. Superficial fascia lies just below the skin and surrounds the entire body.
2. Deep fascia provides structural framework to the skeletal muscles.
3. Subserous fascia supports visceral organs, anchors nerves, and forms walls of blood and lymph vessels.

+ Connective tissue surrounds, supports, connects, compartmentalizes, and protects structures in the body. It provides energy storage through adipose tissue. It transports nutrients and wastes via the blood and lymph, which are *liquid* connective tissue.

+ The deep fascia gives shape to individual muscles. Like layers in a rope, deep fascia surrounds each single muscle fiber, each bundle of fibers that join together to form a single muscle, and also the entire muscle itself. The ends of these deep fascial layers join together and extend beyond the muscle to become the tendons that connect the muscle to the bone.

✦ Fascia spreads tensional strain or ease throughout the body like a global network due to its quality of *tensegrity*. Buckminster Fuller, visionary architect, engineer, inventor, and educator, coined the term *tensegrity*—"tensile integrity"—to describe the ability to spread compressional force. Connective tissues—not the bones—are the guylines that bear most of the structural responsibility for holding the body in a stable upright posture.

✦ Healthy connective tissue can stretch and then return to its original shape. This *elastic recoil,* as it's known, is due to the fundamental spiral formation of the collagen proteins in the connective tissue.[54]

✦ Connective tissue is vascular, meaning it has a lot of blood vessels, except cartilage, which has very little vasculature.

Spinal Rotation: A Primary Pattern

For years in my practice I have noticed rotation patterns in my clients that are affecting them at the core level of their spine. I call this core level rotation a primary rotation pattern. It includes a dominant twist from either right to left or left to right. In general, spinal rotation involves a twist of the "cylinders," or body segments, that comprise the legs, pelvis, and/or thorax. This twisting of the pelvic girdle or the shoulder girdle can then cause vertebral rotation, which can lead to direct or referred pain in the body.

"It must be remembered," said Dr. Rolf, "that the word rotation, like the word curvature, really expresses nothing more frightening than the fact that one muscle (or set of muscles) is pulling more than its structural antagonist is able to balance."[55]

In my 1991 auditing class in Boulder, Colorado, Emmett Hutchins said, "If you have a rotation, something is short. How do you undo that? There is only one way out of it and that is straight through. You only have to go for length. Length is the one archenemy of rotation. You can't have them both."

The Spinal Rotation Pattern

✦ The cylinders of the legs, pelvis, and thorax can turn in different directions.
✦ It is more common for the pelvis to be rotated on the thorax than it is for the thorax to be rotated on the pelvis.

✦ The legs are involved in rotation of the pelvis. Rotation in the legs can hold the pelvis captive.

✦ The rotated girdle will be less organized (that is, less aligned).

✦ Rotation affects each side of the body differently.

✦ A rotation pattern will unwind out of the top and bottom of the less organized girdle.

✦ It may take some time for a core-level rotation to thoroughly resolve.

Indications of Rotation

Generally speaking, in a spinal rotation pattern, if you look at a standing person from the back, one gluteal fold will be higher than the other and the leg on that side will look longer than the other leg. Very often this discrepancy in leg length may be caused by a shortening twist in the connective tissue that affects the joints around it. Less often a bone may actually be anatomically shorter due to an accident or congenital abnormality. In the case of an anatomically shorter bone in the leg, an insert or lift in the shoe might be considered, as such constant discrepancy in leg length will affect the pelvis and the spine all the way to the neck. Other indications of rotation may also be present, including those in the table below.

CHARACTERISTICS OF LONGER AND SHORTER LEG ROTATIONS

LONGER LOOKING LEG	SHORTER LOOKING LEG
Gluteal fold is higher	Gluteal fold is lower
Internal rotation of leg/hip	External rotation of leg/hip
Internal twist in psoas	External twist in psoas
Ilium is forward	Ilium is posterior
Groin is narrow in internal rotation	Groin is wider in external rotation
Internal twist in quadriceps	External twist in quadriceps
Internal twist in knee and ankle	External twist in iliotibial band, knee, and ankle
Foot is more forward or internally rotated	Foot everts or externally rotates
More strain in medial hamstrings	More strain in lateral hamstrings

The Psoas Muscles: Core-Level Players in Spinal Rotation

The psoas muscles are the only muscles that run through the pelvis and connect both halves of the body. The psoas attachment is on the anterior and transverse processes (bony projections that extend from the side of the vertebral bodies) of vertebrae T12–L5. In the front of the body the psoas muscles extend up the spine to the bottom of the diaphragm, just below the center of the rib cage. In the lumbar area, they attach to the internal portion of the vertebral discs as well.

The lower part of the psoas converges with the iliacus muscles, which lie within each side of the pelvis. The tendons of the psoas and iliacus muscles join together and dive underneath each inguinal ligament. They insert on the medial edge of the top of the femur bones on bony protuberances called the lesser trochanters.

Because of their attachment to the vertebrae and intervertebral discs, imbalanced contraction and twist in the psoas muscles can contribute to wear and tear on those discs. That is one of the reasons it is so important to clear rotation patterns at the core of the body. Many people with developing but minor disc problems have found healing and relief through the balanced work of Structural Integration.

Imbalanced Contraction of the Psoas

Having spent years observing and working with spinal rotations, it seems to me that when the psoas muscle on one side of the body contracts, it shortens and pulls the corresponding leg up into the pelvis. This causes that leg to look longer than the other leg from the back side of the body where the gluteal fold is often pulled up higher on the leg of the more contracted psoas. Because of the psoas's origin along the spine and its medial insertion at the lesser trochanter, this contraction of the psoas on one side of the spine also seems to initiate an internal corkscrew-like twist that pulls the spine, pelvis, legs, and feet into rotation.

For example, a shortened psoas on the right side will initiate an internal rotation of the right leg. In its corkscrew-like twist, the rotation pattern will play out on the opposite side of the body as an external rotation, causing the left hip, leg, and foot to turn out. The direction of the twist would be from right to left, with the end of the rotation on the left side of the body. The twist may extend all the way up the spine to the top of the neck, causing the muscles along the left side of the spine to be strained as well.

Lordosis

The psoas muscles can also pull forward away from the spine, causing the lumbar spine to pull forward with them. This causes the pelvis to rotate forward, or anteriorly. This can lead to lordosis, or an exaggerated lumbar curve, and the person's visceral contents may push forward onto the abdominal wall.

When the psoas muscles pull forward away from the spine, they cause strain that can be transmitted through the connective tissues into the secondary thoracic curve of the spine, where the rhomboid muscles lie. If the rhomboid area, which lies along the spine between the scapulae, is strained, then usually the psoas muscles are in trouble as well, and vice versa.

With the pelvis tilted forward, the quadriceps muscles at the top of the front of the legs will also be strained. The quadriceps are responsible for keeping a person with an anterior pelvis from falling forward. In doing so, they become overworked. A person with an anterior pelvis will often have very deep, hard strain in his or her quadriceps groups.

In this situation, release of strain at one end of the spine will create the need for release at the other end of the spine. For example, as the psoas muscles in the pelvic girdle are released, the person will often then experience tightness up in his or her rhomboid area. The upper girdle will then need to be released. This seesaw of strain from one end of the spine to the other occurs naturally as the anterior pelvis returns to a more horizontal position. The "recipe" of Structural Integration supports and addresses such change.

Secondary Rotations

Secondary rotation patterns arising from severe injuries such as sprains or broken bones can be laid on top of a primary rotation and cause a classic rotation pattern to deviate from the norm. In such cases, it is helpful for the practitioner to question a client to bring forth additional information about significant traumas whose effects may be coming into play.

In resolving a compound rotation, in which one rotation pattern is laid on top of another, the body will often go through a process of unwinding. The secondary pattern will usually be the first to unwind, followed by the primary pattern, which will then show itself and be available to be addressed. This would be an example of the body unwinding in layers.

Rotation Patterns Affect the Nervous System

Years ago, during my training with Emmett Hutchins, I asked him whether the autonomic nerves ran through the fibers of each psoas muscle. Emmett replied, "I would say that they are spread out in the membrane that surrounds the psoas. It is in the fascial tissue that the plexus spreads." In other words, autonomic nerves lie in the connective tissues around the psoas muscles.

There are two branches of the autonomic nervous system: the sympathetic "fight or flight" division and the parasympathetic "rest and digest" division. The sympathetic division boosts metabolism, alertness of the body, and preparation for emergency. Its nerves originate along the sides of the spine from the first thoracic vertebra to the second and third lumbar vertebrae, affecting thoracic, lumbar, sacral, and coccygeal areas of the body. The parasympathetic division promotes rest, the uptake of nutrients, and the storage of energy. Its nerves originate in the medulla of the brain stem and sacral segments of the spinal cord.

I have noticed that rotation at the core of the body always involves the psoas muscles and seems to have an effect on both the parasympathetic and sympathetic branches of the autonomic nervous system. I think that because the sacral, lumbar, and solar plexuses lie within or in close proximity to the pelvic basin, a twist in the psoas at the base of the spine will often affect parasympathetic nerves, causing possible digestive, respiratory, and heart rate issues.

As that twist finds its way up the spine via the psoas muscles' connection with the anterior longitudinal ligament on the front side of the spine, the sympathetic nerves along both sides of the spinal erector muscles can become involved as well, causing symptoms like anxiety, panic attacks, and depression to occur.

The all-important cranial nerves III, VII, IX, and X emerge above the cervical area of the neck at the base of the brain stem. This is another area of parasympathetic involvement that can affect heart rate, respiration, and the function of internal organs. A core-level rotation that has moved all the way up the spine can adversely affect those nerves and their areas of enervation.

Dr. Rolf herself spoke about the correlation between psychological issues and structural issues. She knew that psychological ailments could be related to an imbalanced physical counterpart. In describing the changes that are possible through Structural Integration, she stated, "There is an ongoing psychological change as well toward balance, toward serenity, toward a more whole person. The whole person evidences a more apparent, more potent psychic development."[56]

Compressional forces ranging from strain to ease are spread through the body-wide fascial network of connective tissue. This tensegrity quality of the connective tissue allows it to disperse pressures from outside the body. Rotation patterns often have an adverse effect on the connective tissue. Twisting forces of rotation can shorten, adhere, and dehydrate the connective tissue, diminishing its ability to transmit life-force energy. Nerves can become impinged, strength and flexibility of muscles may be impeded, and a lack of circulation may result. This can lead to inflammation, chronic pain, and degeneration of tissues and joints. The process of Structural Integration may assist not only with the resolution of these conditions, it may also lead to the greater organization of the whole person—body, mind, emotion, and spirit.

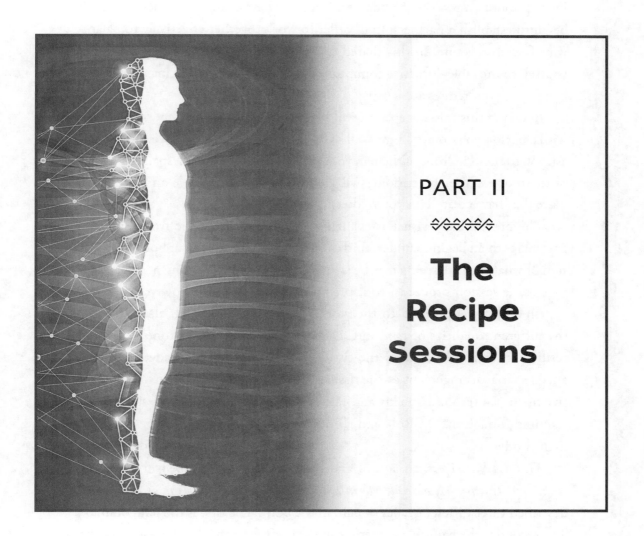

PART II

The
Recipe
Sessions

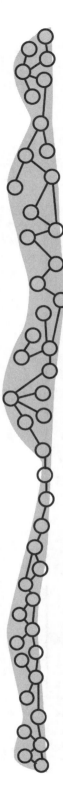

MAXIMIZING THE BENEFITS
OF YOUR TEN SESSIONS

During your first session of Structural Integration, you and your practitioner will begin to establish a partnership in order to work together effectively to balance your fascial structure. In this shared experience, you will each bring the gift of yourself to the table. Effective communication will be essential in maximizing the benefits of your ten-session series.

In taking this initial step, you will likely find yourself in a new environment with a person you do not know well. And this person will even have the nerve to ask you to stand in front of them in your underwear! But don't despair. It's all part of the process. Your practitioner will help you feel comfortable and safe in the place they have created for you to do this work.

The practitioner's visual assessment of your body from the front, side, and back helps them begin to understand the patterns of strain in your body. A discussion of what they are seeing may be shared to launch your working partnership.

As the session proceeds, your practitioner will monitor how your nervous system and fascia respond to the work. Your practitioner will also be noting the different qualities of *tone* and *span* in your tissues. Good tone indicates a resilient chemical balance in the tissue. Good span describes adequately balanced spatial arrangement of the tissue. With good tone and span, the connective tissue can respond quickly and easily to any situation or be at rest when not required for action. Dr. Rolf said, "Both words refer to *balanced structure* in a living body."[1]

Thomas W. Myers, an author and bodyworker widely known for his book *Anatomy Trains: Myofascial Meridians for Manual & Movement Therapists,* described three different types of pain in the body. The first is the pain of injury. The second is the pain that gets stuck in the body. The third is the release of that stored pain.

Practitioners of Structural Integration intend to release the stored pain in the body. They are not trying to create more pain for the client, only to release the pain already stored there. This requires a slow, compassionate process on the part of both practitioner and client.

What can you do to help your practitioner efficiently and effectively release that stored pain in your body?

- ✦ Arrive for your session with viewing clothes, such as underwear, bra, sports bra, or two-piece bathing suit.
- ✦ Focus on relaxing while you receive the work. Let your body drop into the table. Allowing your body to soften and lengthen supports the work, while a contractive response limits the body's ability to release.
- ✦ Breathing through the nose helps the body relax by stimulating the "rest and repair" aspect of the parasympathetic nervous system.
- ✦ Breathe into the area where the practitioner is working to help that area move and stretch. Holding your breath only makes the work more uncomfortable. I tell my clients, "Push my fingers out with your inhalation breath."
- ✦ Speak up! Your feedback is necessary and welcome. Let your practitioner know what is going on. Be your own best advocate.
- ✦ Agree on a way to communicate when you have reached the edge of your ability to relax. This will help your practitioner monitor the pressure.
- ✦ Know that any contraction indicates to your practitioner to lighten the pressure, slow the pace, or pause to let your body integrate.
- ✦ Feel or visualize ease and release in your body when your practitioner takes a moment to pause. When your practitioner begins again, the particular area they were just working with may already have integrated.
- ✦ Follow your practitioner's request for slow movement as directed. Slowly moving the joint in the area being addressed helps the tissue release. The movements of client and practitioner need to be at a similar pace to bring coherence into the work. Such slow, conscious movement supports the parasympathetic nervous system.
- ✦ Let your practitioner know immediately if you experience autonomic symptoms such as light-headedness, increased heart rate, nausea, or sweating. These indicate that the work needs to be slowed way down or stopped to let your body integrate.

Enjoy your process of transformation and integration. Give it your best go! Let yourself be moved by this work, and follow your practitioner's suggestions.

May your investment in Structural Integration reap huge rewards for you on many levels. Blessings to you!

Before the First Session

Before you begin, write down all your current symptoms and conditions that you would like to resolve. Formulate your goals and intentions. Doing this will enhance the benefits of your ten-series investment.

The body has a great capacity to shift with this work. You may notice changes immediately upon standing after the session, or you may experience them as an accumulating effect throughout the series. Toward the end of your ten-session series, the majority of the ailments on your list may be completely forgotten or significantly improved. Each person's experience of the work will be unique according to their own body's needs and personal history.

Because of the connection between body, mind, emotion, and spirit, you might consider not only physical goals but also personal goals. This work is a springboard for creating major positive change. It can usher in the next level of who you are becoming. With that in mind, what is it in your life that you would like to bring in or accomplish at this time?

Drink plenty of water before your first session and every session thereafter. Good hydration will help your body release more easily and clear toxins more quickly. You might also consider supplementing with vitamin C before your session. Vitamin C can help strengthen the walls of the capillaries and prevent them from breaking, which causes bruising. Vitamin C is also a powerful antioxidant and helps with the formation and maintenance of connective tissue.

Working with the Energetics
of the Line after Each Session

The organization of the body in each session builds an energetic capacity to experience the movement of life-force energy through the Line. Because of this, I share an experience of the Line with the client at the end of each session. In this way, I am educating clients in how they *can* consciously participate in the movement of life-force energy in their body. It can be very exciting for them. I teach people that it *is* possible to do that and encourage them to pay attention to the experience of their Line in an ongoing manner outside of our Structural Integration sessions. Working with the movement of the electromagnetic life-force energy is very qi gong–like, and some people relate to it more easily than others. As a person's body becomes more organized, so does a person's capacity to experience the energetics of the Line. The movement of life-force energy is a subtle experience and requires repetition after *each* session for that capacity to be reinforced in a person. Such repetition helps to support a person's learning curve.

To help people find the balanced stacking of their major body segments in a standing position, I will often have them stand close to a wall with their feet slightly away from it, their hips barely touching it, and their head drawn back slightly so their ears are over the center of their shoulders if there is a forward tendency of the head. In this way, the person's major segments can be stacked, so that their center of gravity aligns around their central vertical axis. Gentle guidance of body segments into a more optimal position may be necessary. My goal is for clients to be able to find the optimal stacking of their body segments on their own while they are standing and sitting and then be able to experience the running of the electromagnetic life-force energy through their Line. Reinforcement of the person's experience of their Line at the end of each session helps to build the client's confidence and ability to experience it. I recommend practicing finding the Line and noticing how the experience changes between each session and beyond.

♟ Exercise: Finding the Standing Line

To experience your standing Line, stand with your feet only about 3 inches apart. Your heels should not be farther apart than the sitting bones of your hips. (If your heels are spread wider, your sacrum will not be able to move freely—and as we've noted, movement is life.) Feel your weight in your feet. Rock forward onto the balls of your feet, then backward onto your heels. Find the place in the center of the two. Let your weight settle right in front of your anklebones. That's the center of your feet. It's the place where you can drop into and be supported. Let yourself drop into that place. That's good.

Bring your attention to your head. Feel the tops of your ears. Imagine drawing a line from the top of each ear to the top of your head. The place where those lines would intersect is the exact top of your head. That is where *up* is. Dr. Rolf used to say that people don't know where *up* is, but now you have found it. Touch it.

Your Line extends from the Earth up through the center of the feet and legs and runs along the front side of the spine, extending out through the top of the head, your *up*, into the heavens. Breath is the pump that moves the life-force energy of the Earth and heavens through the conduit of your body, energizing all of your major systems. Let's breathe along this Line. With each breath, visualize Earth energy moving into the bottoms of your feet. Draw it through the center of your feet, up the center of your legs, and along the front of your spine. Breath doesn't stop at the top of your chest; continue drawing your breath up through the center of your neck and head. At the top of your head, let the energy shower out into the energy field that surrounds your body. Breathing in this way creates a quality of lift throughout your body. You may feel a tingling sensation as the subtle life-force energy begins to move in you.

Similarly, heavenly energy can move down into your body through the top of your head toward the bottoms of your feet. I use an inhalation to pull energy from the celestial sun and stars into my body through the top of my head. Then, with my exhalation, I send that energy down into every cell of my body through my Line of connection.

Both energies are necessary for the body. They are the yin and the yang, the negative and the positive, the feminine and the masculine. All matter on our Earth is a combination of yin and yang energy or qi. Each seeks the other to create balance. Together, they create a whole.

⚘ Exercise: Finding the Sitting Line

To find your sitting Line, sit in a chair with your feet flat on the floor and your head held upright. Check your posture for alignment: your lumbar curve should be in place, and your shoulders should rest with ease on your rib cage, which should be stacked above your pelvis. Your core muscles hold you upright.

As you did in the exercise above to find your standing Line, bring your awareness to the top of your head, where *up* is. Then bring your awareness to the bottom of that connection, which now, in a seated position, is at your tailbone. In this position, your central nervous system is alert and aware. See if you can notice the energy moving through you. Try this at your desk or computer as you work. It can change your life.

You can connect with your Line anytime, in any position. You can even connect to your Line while you are moving by maintaining awareness of your feet as the base of support for every action. That awareness is the foundation to experiencing your Line of connection. It is a place of personal power. It is where we connect into the *being* and *doing* of life. The quality of our life is affected by the quality of our connection. It's about partnering up with larger spheres of energy. We call this "being on our Line." When we are on our Line, we are not alone. As Emmett said, through the Line, we connect into the transcendent.

Self-Care after Each Session

The work of Structural Integration helps to balance soft tissues that have gotten disorganized in the body. The release of such tissues and their accumulated toxins may cause the body to feel sore after a session. Some simple self-care practices can help relieve soreness and help your body integrate the work.

+ **Take a short walk.** A ten-minute walk immediately after your Structural Integration session will help your body integrate its changes in relationship to gravity.

+ **Submerge in a detoxifying bath.** Structural Integration work can release toxins from your tissues, with possible side effects including dizziness, headache, nausea, body ache, fever, or flu-like symptoms. If the toxins are not removed from your body, they can move back into the bloodstream into deeper layers of the connective tissues. Take a detox bath for *three days in a row*: The first bath is taken shortly after your session, as soon as possible, or at least within six hours. The second bath is early in the morning of the following day. The third bath is in the evening of the third day following your session. See page 40 for details on detox baths.

+ **Use arnica gel to relieve soreness.** If you are still experiencing any soreness after your detox baths, rub some arnica gel into the painful area. Arnica increases circulation and reduces inflammation, which relieves pain.

+ **Try a steam bath or sauna.** Steam rooms and saunas, particularly the far-infrared saunas (see page 128), can expedite the release of toxins that have gotten stirred up from the bodywork.

+ **Increase your water intake for the entire series of sessions**. Water rehydrates the connective tissues and helps flush out toxins. A good rule of thumb is to drink half of your body weight in ounces of water per day. Coffee is considered to be dehydrating, so add 2 cups of water for every cup of coffee you drink.

✦ **Increase your protein intake for the entire series of sessions.** Extra protein will support the formation of new connective tissues during this time of reorganization in your body.

✦ **Consider herbal anti-inflammatories for the entire series of sessions.** These natural products can relieve inflammation throughout the body, helping to minimize soreness and ease the passage of strain from your body. I prefer turmeric products.

✦ **Don't challenge your body right after a session.** This is a really important time to listen to your body and take precautions because you are new and different. Your proprioception has changed. You may want to make different movement choices after the session to allow the work to integrate. As stated above, walking is typically a great way to integrate after a session.

The Detox Bath

At its simplest, a detoxifying bath is a warm but not exceedingly hot bath to which 2 cups of Epsom salts and 2 cups of baking soda have been added. Soak in the bath for a minimum of twenty minutes.

Epsom salts is a form of magnesium sulfate, which is itself comprised of magnesium and sulfur. The magnesium soaks into the muscles and helps them relax. The sulfur helps reduce inflammation and pain in the joints. Whether you are dealing with sore, inflamed joints or tight muscles, magnesium sulfate has a powerful beneficial effect.

The baking soda helps neutralize the acidic toxins that are stirred up by bodywork or strenuous activity.

While you are soaking, keep all of your body parts well submerged, particularly the ones that were just addressed in your bodywork session. Drink 10 to 12 ounces of water while you are soaking to help flush out toxins and rehydrate, and be sure to shower off when you are done to remove salts, which can be drying to the skin.

If bathing makes your skin dry, try adding powdered oats as an emollient. Just blend 1 to 2 cups of rolled oats in a blender until you have a fine powder and add it to the bathwater.

I have used this soothing, revitalizing detox bath for years as a practitioner. It helps ease any strain in my body.

Emotional Release

Energy in the form of mental and emotional stress can get stuck in the tissues of the body. Bodywork can facilitate the release of these "stuck" mental and emotional patterns, stirring up old memories and emotions. The movement of such energy can be surprising and disturbing. If it happens, don't worry about it. It is a natural cleansing process and an opportunity to let go. Let these emotions and memories move like television images in front of you. They simply represent energy in the body that needs to be released.

Relaxation and deep breathing during your sessions can reduce the intensity of strong sensations and emotions. If you can relax into the pain and allow yourself to fully experience it, those sensations can change into a feeling of release. When you bring your breath, awareness, willingness, and love to an area of pain, it changes. Tissues have the opportunity to clear and reorganize on physical *and* energetic levels. In this way, Structural Integration is a purification process that helps people get lighter and brighter.

During your Structural Integration series, your body and psyche will transform gradually. Personal evolution unfolds in spiraling layers. We don't change all at once. It is important to be gentle with yourself and cut yourself slack during your Structural Integration series. Let the people close to you know that you're going through a significant process of change.

Do not make any major life changes during the time when you are receiving your ten sessions. During this work, your body will change not only physically but also mentally and emotionally. Give yourself time to integrate such changes before making any major life decisions.

Joseph Heller, a respected student of Dr. Rolf and a former president of the Rolf Institute, is the founder of Hellerwork Structural Integration and an authority on the emotions and their effects on different parts of the body. Heller's insightful themes added another level of depth to the work. The discussions of the sessions that follow each begin with his themes and comments and include his movement exercises and renderings of some illustrations from the 1990 Hellerwork *Client's Handbook.*

To delve deeper into the Hellerwork philosophy and themes, or to find out how to become a Hellerwork practitioner, go to the Hellerwork website at www .Hellerwork.com. Please note that there are other certified schools of Structural Integration that have distinct focuses. They can be found at www.theiasi.net.

SESSION ONE
Inspiration

The Theme of the First Session

Joseph Heller described the theme of the first session as "inspiration." As he said, "The meaning of the word 'inspiration' is 'draw in spirit': inspiration is not only to inhale oxygen, but it is also to be filled with—or to be in touch with—spirit."[2] Breath is our prime connection with life force. The first session can be an inspiration for being able to breathe deeply and to fully give and receive love.

The spirit of the first session is of being reborn. The psychological Hellerwork connection here is the reawakening of an enthusiasm for life—of discovering the possibility of newfound freedom in body, mind, emotion, and spirit. The potential of "being" is stirred.

Emmett Hutchins, my first teacher of Dr. Rolf's work, told me that the mood of the first hour is, "Wow! That was wonderful. I've never had anything like that before. Can I get more?"

Dr. Rolf's Words Related to the First Session

"When the position of the ribs is changed, breathing changes. . . . Now there isn't anyone that knows so little about biological chemistry that he doesn't understand that getting more air into the lungs and getting it moving faster is going to change the chemistry of every cell in the body. So in a first Rolfing hour, we have started changing the chemistry of every cell in the body in the first ten minutes. . . . All of a sudden the skin becomes pink; the skin may be a little more moist—the glands of the skin are working."[3]

Practitioner Goals
for the First Session

+ Develop awareness of client's baseline structure.
+ Begin to build a working relationship with the client.
+ Open up breathing capacity.
+ Lengthen the front of the body.
+ Begin to release restrictions in the pelvic and shoulder girdles.
+ Begin to release the superficial fascia.
+ Begin to free the legs.
+ Horizontalize and mobilize the pelvis.
+ Introduce the client to their Line. Acquaint the client with where the top of their head and feet align in relation to the gravitational field.

Areas Addressed

The front of the body will be longer after this session, which means that the back will need to be lengthened in the second session. This is the beginning of freeing strain in the rib cage, shoulder girdle, legs, hips, neck, and back. Breathing capacity will improve. The client's weight, when standing, may shift onto the heels. As the weight bearing down on the feet shifts, the rib cage may lift.

A client of mine who was a medical doctor and athlete excitedly reported what he felt was a 25 percent increase in his breathing capacity after his first session. As a result, he sailed through his cycling competition the next day with increased ease and stamina.

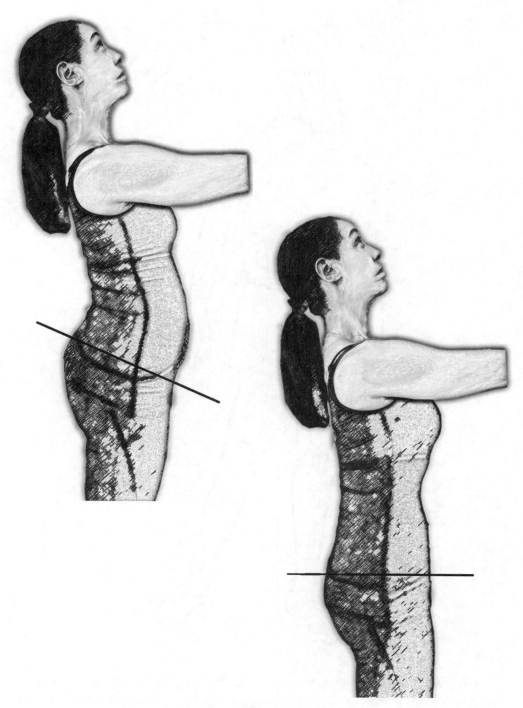

✦ Fig. 2.1. (A) Anterior (tilted forward) pelvis; (B) horizontal pelvis.

These illustrations were produced by and used with kind permission of
Andreini McPherson-Husbands and Andreina Shelton.

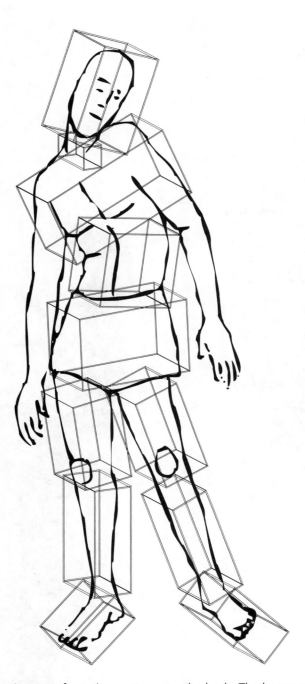

◆ Fig. 2.2. The impact of rotation patterns on the body. The boxes represent body segments—or as Dr. Rolf called them, an aggregate of blocks—that are out of alignment due to a rotational pattern, thus throwing off the center of gravity of the body.

This drawing was adapted by Carolyn Cameron from the Hellerwork *Client's Handbook* and used with kind permission of Hellerwork International, LLC.

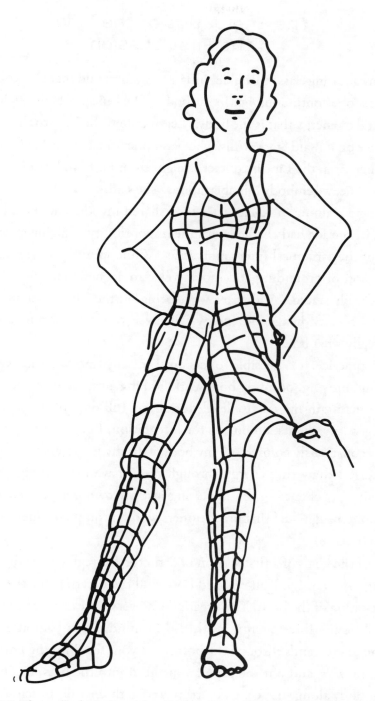

◆ Fig. 2.3. The pull of tension through the connective tissue "body stocking."

This drawing was adapted by Carolyn Cameron from the Hellerwork *Client's Handbook* and used with kind permission of Hellerwork International, LLC.

The Energetics of the Line
in the First Session

During my auditing class in Boulder in 1991, Emmett said that Dr. Rolf described the Line as "one continuous *now* in the body." The Line passes through the center of the spiral of energy that is the body. "Learn to love the Line to the point where you can live on it," said Stacy Mills, who was a phenomenal teacher in my auditing class. "Inherent in the Line is contact straight from Earth to heaven. If we are not using our Line, we embody our aberrations," she said.

During a training in Kauai in 2012, I shared my ideas about the Line with Emmett, whom Ida had charged with the responsibility of giving meaning to the "recipe" of the Structural Integration series. While speaking with him about the phenomenon of grounding and moving electromagnetic energy in my body, I enthusiastically stated, "And that's what being on the Line is about—it's about running the electromagnetic energy wherever you are!" Emmett responded, "That's really what it is."

With practice, it is possible to feel our Line anytime, whether we are standing, sitting, moving, or doing bodywork. Taking a moment to get on my Line helps me maintain my energy level during my full days of work with clients. When I give my clients a moment for integration, I get on Line, breathe, and recharge, consciously connecting my body with the larger energy fields around me. Because I draw that energy through me, I have more energy available as I work with my clients—I am not using just my own personal energy for the work. Emmett suggested that practitioners who stay on their Line won't become fatigued. It's true!

One of the goals of a first session of Structural Integration is to increase the breathing capacity. Dr. Rolf realized how vital the breath is for the physiological functioning of the body. The breath is also very necessary for the movement of our subtle life-force energy. With this in mind, focus your attention along your Line that extends through the bottom of your feet into the Earth, through your central axis, and out the top of your head into the heavens. Invite this qi into your body along your central vertical axis with the full conscious inhalation and exhalation of your breath. Long, slow breathing in this manner engages the movement of the diaphragm, which is important for the movement of life-force energy in the body.

Self-Care for the Client
after the First Session

Follow the suggestions for self-care that are outlined beginning on page 39, particularly taking a short walk immediately after your session and taking your first detox bath within six hours. Remember to drink plenty of water.

Movement Awareness for
the Client after the First Session

Breath has the potential to move in all directions in the body. When you breathe in, your rib cage should be able to fully expand—that is, from front to back, from side to side, and from top to bottom. This ability to fully breathe will help oxygenate all the cells and tissues of your body.

Bring your awareness to this movement. While lying on your back or standing, place a hand on each side of your ribs and fully expand your breath in each direction. Are your ribs able to move freely? Follow your breath up and down your spine. Are there any still spots where your breath cannot move?

Breath has the ability to move through the center of the neck, up through the center of the head, and out the top into the energy field of the body. Do you allow yourself to fully breathe this way? Are you aware of your breath moving through the center of your head, or does it stop at the top of your neck?

When you breathe all the way through the center of your head, that movement rocks your head into better alignment over the central axis of the body. The movement will look like a little bobble. Moving your breath with awareness through the center of your head energizes important energy centers in your body. It is a thorough way to breathe. See if you can move your breath through your neck and then through the center of your head and out the top. Surrender yourself to full inhalations and exhalations, without forcing either.

Between the First
and Second Sessions

Because the psyche and body are so connected, the practitioner's work around the rib cage may cause feelings to surface during or after the session. Often freeing the breath provokes a reawakened enthusiasm for life; however, the first session can also stir up repressed emotions like sadness.

Did the first session of Structural Integration cause any feelings to come up for you? Did this surprise you? How did you handle those emotions? Was it okay for you to feel the feelings, or did you try to stifle them? This might be an opportunity for you to clear some of those feelings on the mental and emotional levels and get them "off your chest."

SESSION TWO

Standing on Your Own Two Feet

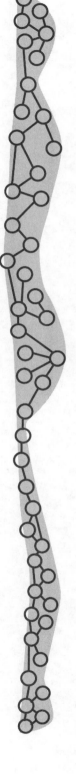

The Theme of the Second Session

Joseph Heller described the theme of this session as "standing on your own two feet." "Independence requires support. Without the support of the ground, our legs would be useless. Independence does not mean we cannot depend on anyone else. On the contrary, we need stability in order to receive support. In the physical world, the ground is our ultimate support and it is through our support and through our feet and legs that we experience it. In what ways do you stand on your own two feet? In your desire to be independent, do you still allow support? In this session we consider the integration of independence and support."[4]

Dr. Rolf's Words Related to the Second Session

"Balance in the body begins with feet, for the basic work of foot and ankle is to offer a reliable base by which the upper body can relate to the horizontal plane of the earth. . . . Only by bringing peace 'from the ground up' can problems higher in the body be understood."[5]

"It should sink into the ground," Emmett Hutchins expanded. "An alive foot hits the floor like an animal's paw. The movement should be really open, not just heel-toe. Going barefoot wakes up the intrinsic muscles of the feet."

Practitioner Goals for the Second Session

+ Ground the work begun in the first session.
+ Balance the three arches of each foot.
+ Begin to establish functional horizontal hinges in the feet, ankles, and knees.

✦ Create space in the feet. Build a foundation for the heels to go into
  the Earth.
✦ Free the fibula.
✦ Distribute the body weight appropriately over the arches
  of the feet.
✦ Lengthen and balance the front, back, and sides of the legs.
✦ Lengthen the back to bring about a balance to the front.

Areas Addressed

The second session addresses the superficial musculature and fascia of the feet,
ankles, knees, legs, and back. We begin to establish optimal balance in the feet and
legs through work that brings the knee and ankle joints to a more horizontal position. Corrections are made in foot alignment, stance, and walking, if needed. The
psychological Hellerwork connection addresses the establishment of a firm foundation underneath us through proper alignment and support of our feet and legs.
The energetic potential of connection of our feet into the ground/Earth energy is
established. We then carry that connection into the Line.

"The goal of the second session is to build a foundation for the heels to go
into the Earth," according to Emmett Hutchins. "Energy should flow through
the heels and up through the back to the top of the head. It involves work on the
plantar fascia, on the bottom of the feet. We are talking to the core all the way to
the top of the head."

Emmett also noted, "This session can shake up your whole sense of reality. It
affects the core-level belief system stuff."

The Energetics of the Line
in the Second Session

In 2010, Clinton Ober, Stephen T. Sinatra, and Martin Zucker published a book
called *Earthing*, with a foreword by James L. Oschman. The authors put forward the ideas of credible scientists who consider the Earth to be, as Oschman
put it, "one gigantic anti-inflammatory, sleep booster, and energizer all wrapped
up in one."[6]

The authors propose that the Earth's surface is covered with a vast reservoir

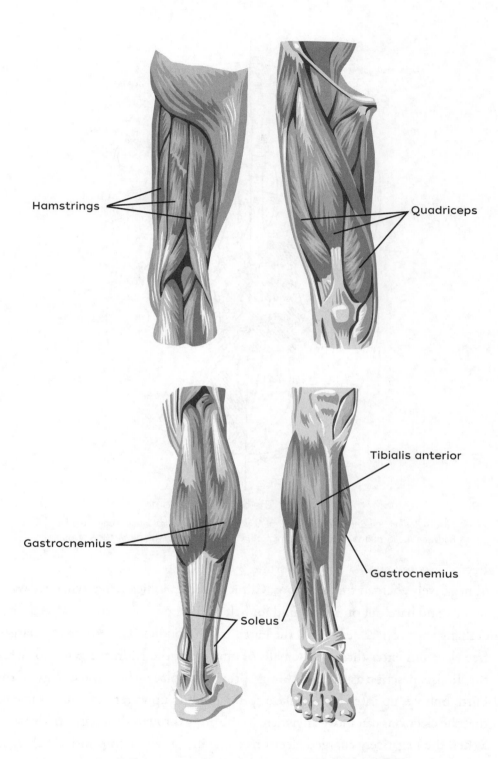

✦ Fig. 2.4. The muscles of the feet and legs, anterior and posterior.
From URRRA/Shutterstock.com.

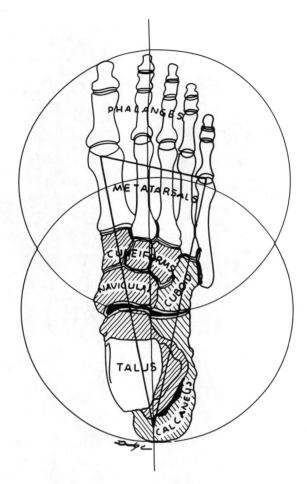

✦ Fig. 2.5. The bones of the foot.

From *Rolfing: Reestablishing the Natural Alignment and Structural Integration of the Human Body for Vitality and Well-Being* by Ida P. Rolf, Ph.D. Reprinted with permission of publisher.

of negatively charged free electrons. Clinical studies indicate that when we walk, sit, or stand barefoot on the ground for half an hour or so, it activates an electrical exchange between the energy of the Earth and our bodies. The negatively charged free electrons enter through the balls of our feet at the Kidney 1 point, or what the Taoists describe as the "Bubbling Spring," the place where the energy of the Earth bubbles up into the feet like a spring bubbles up water. Oschman suggests that the electrons can move anywhere in the body through the connective tissues. When the negatively charged electrons come in contact with positively charged free radicals, they neutralize them. Free radicals create inflammation in the body. Benefits of this energy exchange include the reduction or elimination of chronic

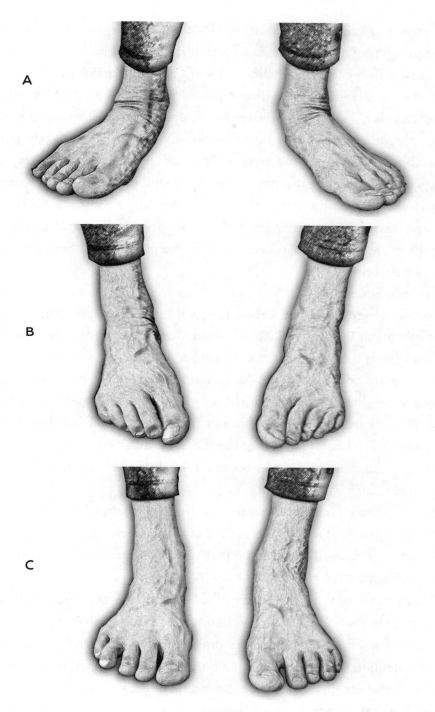

♦ Fig 2.6. (A) Weight on the inner arches (knock-knees); (B) weight on
the outer arches (bowlegs); (C) weight balanced on the feet (aligned legs).

These illustrations were produced and used with kind permission of
Andreini McPherson-Husbands and Andreina Shelton.

inflammation, autoimmune diseases, chronic pain, stress, fatigue, anxiety, and premature aging. The implications are potentially enormous. Scientists are even stating that inflammation may be the result of an electron deficiency in the body.[7]

In a 1997 article in *Footwear News,* the late Dr. William Rossi, a Massachusetts podiatrist, wrote, "The sole of the foot is richly covered with some 1,300 nerve endings per square inch. That's more than found on any other part of the body of comparable size. Why so many nerve endings concentrated there? To keep us 'in touch' with the earth, the real physical world around us. . . . The foot is the vital link between the person and the earth. The paws of all animals are equally rich in nerve endings. . . . The earth is covered with an electromagnetic layer. . . . Every living thing, including human beings, draws energy from this field through its feet, paws, or roots."[8]

As Ober, Sinatra, and Zucker note, "In developed societies, in particular, we have lost our electrical roots. Our bare feet, with their rich network of nerve endings, rarely touch the ground."[9] Since World War II, our modern day shoes have been made with insulating materials of rubber, plastic, and petrochemical compounds that are nonconductive.[10] Sadly, Dr. Rossi stated, "The bottoms of our footwear are so thick or heavy that the sole of the foot is virtually 'deadened.'"[11] David Wolfe, Earth activist, author, and founder of The Fruit Tree Planting Foundation, incriminates shoes as one of the "most destructive culprits of inflammation and autoimmune diseases because they disconnect us from the healing energy of the Earth."[12]

"Shoes and sandals used to be made from leather processed from hides. When moist, leather is a conductive material. The original lightweight soft sole, heel-less simple moccasin is possibly the closest we have come to an 'ideal' shoe and it dates back more than 14,000 years ago."[13]

The electrons of the Earth's energy field have wave-particle duality, meaning that they can be particles or waves. We know from quantum physics that intention can cause these subatomic particles to organize. The mystic in me believes that through intention we can activate the running of Earth energy through the body, regardless of whether or not we are grounding directly on the Earth. I "invite" this Earth energy to enter my body through the bottoms of my feet. My body has learned to resonate with this energy. I feel the tingling of these waves of energy as they move through me. You can too.

Try it. Set aside the inner critic, the inner judge, the one who has it all figured out. Put a smile on your face, and invite that energy in. Use your breath like a pump to move it. Enjoy! It is a feast for your cells and a great Line exercise after your second session.

Self-Care for the Client
after the Second Session

Follow the suggestions for self-care that are outlined beginning on page 39, particularly taking a short walk immediately after your session and taking your first detox bath within six hours. Remember to drink plenty of water.

Movement Awareness for the Client
after the Second Session

Notice your new stance now that your practitioner has shown you proper alignment through your feet. The optimal position for your feet is pointed straight, parallel to each other. Your body weight should drop down your legs into the front of your anklebones. You should carry your weight in the middle of your feet, in front of your ankles, not on your heels or the balls of your feet.

Pay attention to how you walk. Your weight should flow evenly through the center of your foot along the line of the second toe, passing through the heel, instep, ball, and then toe as the foot gets ready to lift up again. Allow your walk to be soft and fluid. Practice walking with this new information. Don't try to alter your gait or stance until you have had the second session of bodywork to remove any existing myofascial strain patterns. To do so would be like putting a maladaptive pattern on top of a preexisting maladaptive pattern.

Take a look at your shoes. If they are worn unevenly on the inside or outside edges, this would be an ideal time to get a new pair. New shoes will support your new foundation. Strapless shoes and flip-flops are definitely *not* recommended, as they create abnormal strain patterns in the feet.

If you have problem arches or if your feet have tracked in or out, try this simple exercise to engage the muscles in your lower legs and ankles to pull up your arches for proper standing and walking: Stand with your feet parallel to each other and your back upright. Keeping your back straight, slowly bend both knees to bring the center of the kneecaps directly over your second toes. Then rise slowly back to your standing position, maintaining awareness of your ankles and knees to be sure that they don't roll in or out. Notice whether this movement engages any muscles that were not previously engaging.

Notice whether you have one hip or arm that is dominant in leading when you walk. That may indicate a rotation pattern in the shoulder or pelvic girdle. Just noticing is fine for now.

Massage your feet, ankles, and lower legs. Then, when you stand and walk, notice how your feet make better contact with the surface beneath you. Massaging your feet, ankles, and lower legs will assist with the softening and lengthening of those connective tissues. It will help your body move more freely and allow your feet to be more malleable with the surface you are walking on.

Between the
Second and Third Sessions

Structural Integration may stir up memories and emotions that are stored in the connective tissues. This presents an opportunity for them to heal. "We know that all negative energy tightens and shortens the body," said Emmett. "Dr. Rolf gave Moshe Feldenkrais the credit for discovering that negative emotions shrink the flexors of the body."

"The recipe tells us to stop getting small," he continued. "Stop protecting. Stop consolidating. Stop being a force against the universe from the inside. Join the party." The second hour of Structural Integration is saying, "Stand in the field."

The legs can be a place where we store concerns about grounding and security. Joseph Heller suggested that the second session leads us to ponder issues around our personal stability and support. After the second session, notice how stable you feel physically, mentally, emotionally, financially, and in your relationships. Consider ways to bring increased stability into some aspects of your life that need support. Allow yourself to be supported.[14]

SESSION THREE
Reaching Out

The Theme of the Third Session

Joseph Heller's theme for the third session is "reaching out." He said, "In the context of this session reaching out has two meanings. The first meaning is that of making contact, giving and receiving, asserting yourself, and asking for what you need. The second meaning involves aggression and the expression of anger. It is no accident that 'arms' is another word for weapons. The arms are, therefore, the embodiment of both meanings. The sides support the arms in reaching out, and are expressive of support in relationship to others, as in 'stand by my side.' Do you reach out to others? Is it easier for you to ask for support or to lend it? After the second session, which is about self-sufficiency and being grounded on your own two feet, you now have a solid foundation from which to reach out and make contact with people."[15]

Dr. Rolf's Words Related to the Third Session

The goal of this session is the "freeing of the core structures from the drag of the girdles by lengthening the lateral aspects of the body. Imbalances in the body are now most apparent in its lateral aspects. These must be lengthened by working under the shoulder girdle, up the ribs and along the pelvic girdle."[16]

Practitioner Goals for the Third Session

+ Release tension in the shoulders, arms, and sides of the body.
+ Lengthen the sides of the body between the pelvic girdle and the shoulder girdle.
+ Bring vertical alignment to the sides of the body.

◆ Separate the structures of the front from the back.

◆ Create the space for the twelfth rib to "breathe."

Areas Addressed

The areas addressed include the rib cage, the outside of the legs, and the sides of the body, arms, neck, and back. The focus of this session is to align the sides of the torso vertically. The establishment of this third-session Line can be compared to that of aligning a side seam of clothing more vertically.

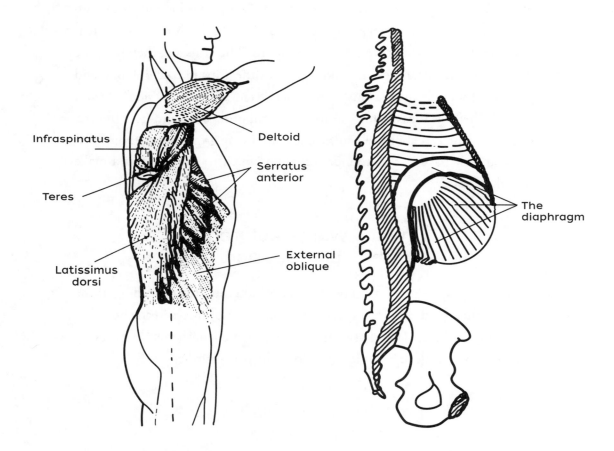

◆ Fig. 2.7. The musculature of the side of the body.

From *Rolfing: Reestablishing the Natural Alignment and Structural Integration of the Human Body for Vitality and Well-Being* by Ida P. Rolf, Ph.D. Reprinted with permission of publisher.

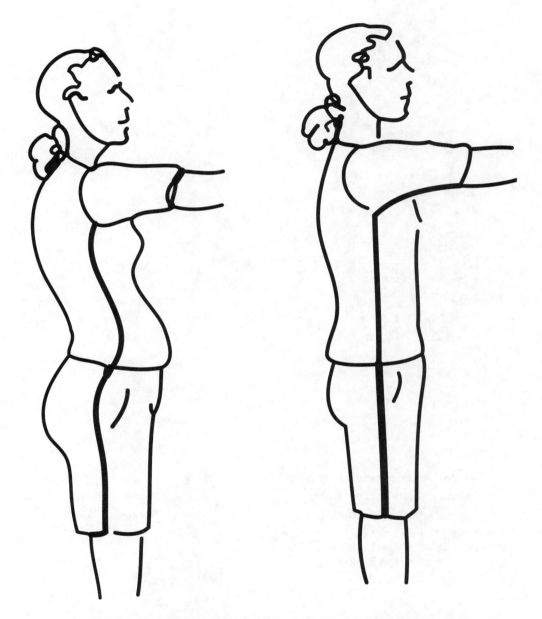

✦ Fig. 2.8. The "side seam" of the body before and after alignment.

This drawing was adapted by Carolyn Cameron from the Hellerwork *Client's Handbook* and used with kind permission of Hellerwork International, LLC.

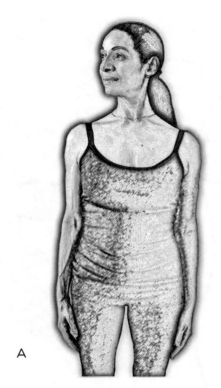

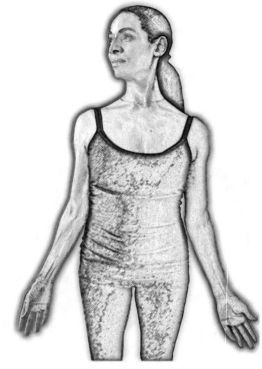

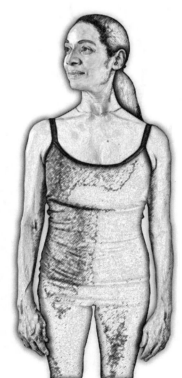

◆ Fig. 2.9. Arm positions: (A) rotated inward; (B) rotated outward; (C) most functional.

These illustrations were produced by and used with kind permission of Andreini McPherson-Husbands and Andreina Shelton.

The Energetics of the Line
in the Third Session

⚮ Exercise: Expanding with Your Breath

As you stand on your Line, bring your awareness to your breath. See how fully you can let your rib cage expand with respiration. Can you feel movement of your breath from your feet to the top of your head? As you learned in the first session, breath does not stop at the top of the chest but moves up the neck, through the center of the head, and out the top of the head into the energy field surrounding the body. Breath can also move from the very front of the chest to the back of the back. And now that we have completed the third-session Line, you may feel the sides of your body expand more fully as you breathe.

Think of your breath as a pump that moves Earth energy from your feet all the way through the top of your head. Your breath can also move heavenly energy down through the top of your head to your feet. In this way, heavenly and earthly energies run from above and below. These fields of energy can support the human body much more than we "moderns" might think.

Take another big breath. Let it move from your feet to the top of your head and out into your energy field. Fill up your rib cage three-dimensionally, from front to back, side to side, and top to bottom. How does that feel? Do you sense your breath moving fully in each of those directions? Are there any places where your breath is not moving freely? Notice that.

By the end of the third session, we have addressed the outer envelope of the body, working with the superficial fascia of the front, back, and now the sides of the body. The third session prepares the body for work at the core-level layers, which will follow. The inner Line needs to be opened up, which we will do in our fourth session.

Self-Care for the Client
after the Third Session

Follow the suggestions for self-care that are outlined beginning on page 39, particularly taking a short walk immediately after your session and taking your first detox bath within six hours. Remember to drink plenty of water.

Movement Awareness for the Client
after the Third Session

Lateral Breathing

The third session is an important breathwork session. After this session, your rib cage is free to expand sideways; we call this lateral breathing. Ideally, breath moves in six directions in the body—that is, from front to back, side to side, and up and down. Take a breath and fully fill your rib cage, letting it move in these different ways. As you go about your day after the third session, maintain awareness of your breathing.

The Sitting Line

Joseph Heller said, "One of the hardest things to convince people of is that their arms were meant to hang."[17] Shoulders do not need to be intentionally pulled back on the torso for "correct" posture. Neither should they slump forward, pulling the head forward with them. Rather, the shoulders should hang naturally over the rib cage, like a coat hanger, with the arms able to swing freely. There's no need to force them back. When strain is taken out of the tissues related to the shoulder girdle, the shoulders will happily lie on and be supported by the bones of the ribs below them.

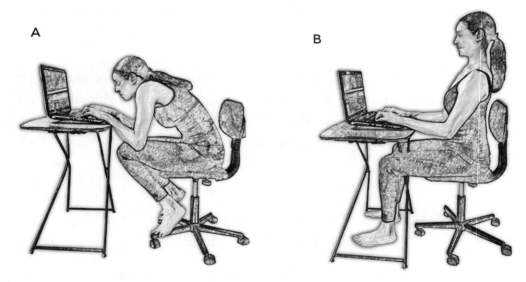

A

B

✦ Fig. 2.10. (A) Incorrect slouching; (B) correct sitting Line.

These illustrations were produced by and used with kind permission of
Andreini McPherson-Husbands and Andreina Shelton.

⚹ Exercise: The Sitting Line

Sit upright in a chair with your feet flat on the floor. Allow your lower back to have a natural gentle curve. We call this the lumbar curve. Notice your *up*—that is, the place at the top of your head centered between your ears.

Now let's see the effect of slouching on the body. Let your lumbar curve slump forward and see how that causes your head and shoulders to fall forward as well. Shrug your shoulders upward and notice how easily your shoulders can migrate up toward your ears. This movement of the shoulders toward the ears creates strain in the shoulders, neck, back, and head, as that position forces them to fall forward. Many office workers take on this disorganized posture. Start today to become more conscious of sitting on your Line at your desk.

Now, get on your sitting Line again, with your feet flat on the floor, your lumbar curve in, and your shoulders upright and in line with your ears. Lift through the energetic central line that runs through your spine and out the top of your head. Notice how clear your awareness is in this organized sitting position. Sitting in this position energizes the central nervous system. Shrug your shoulders once more, and feel how difficult it is to lift your shoulders up to your ears while sitting upright on your Line. They do not move upward as easily as they did when you were sitting in a slouched position.

Sitting on your Line with lift through the top of your head will help your shoulder girdle stay relaxed and balanced on your rib cage. It also energizes your body with an alert awareness. Your arms will be able to hang freely. They don't need to be held up by your neck, back, and shoulders. This is an efficient way to sit and work. As you sit on your Line, just remember to lift through the top of your head.

Arm Alignment

People carry their arms in different ways. Sometimes a person's shoulders will pull back and their arms will turn out. Sometimes the shoulders will come forward and the arms will turn in. The palms sometimes face forward, sometimes inward, and sometimes backward. Which is correct? It seems to be a point in question within different bodywork modalities.

In Structural Integration, the most efficient arm position is considered to be the one where the shoulder girdle is not rotated externally, with the palms facing forward. That would be similar to the feet being turned out with an external rotation of the pelvic girdle. Instead, proper alignment has the palms facing backward and elbows pointed out. This position allows the shoulders to be used in their full range of motion.

Become aware of how your arms are hanging at this moment. However they are hanging is fine. It is not helpful to force them into any other position. With awareness of how you use your arms and as you receive more Structural Integration work, your shoulder girdle will naturally align toward its optimal position.

Between the
Third and Fourth Sessions

The third-session work in the shoulder girdle can help release chronically held attitudes that limit our ability to reach out for what we want and allow us to receive. Joseph Heller suggests that before the fourth session you should notice when you are having a hard time reaching for what you want and when you find yourself holding back either affection or anger and frustration.[18] During those moments, check to see if you are carrying any tension in your arms or along the sides of your body. Notice how that feels. Bring attention and ease to those areas, as needed.

SESSION FOUR
Control and Surrender

The Theme of the Fourth Session

Joseph Heller described the theme of the fourth session as "control and surrender." He said:

> One of the first acts of self-control that we are asked to perform as a child is toilet training, requiring control of the muscles of the bottom of the core. After that, personal control can become equated with holding things inside the body: "keeping it together," not crying, not letting anything out that "shouldn't" be out.
>
> Surrender is something the enemy did after the war; in other words, giving up, failing. Nonetheless, "control" is not necessarily rigid or suppressive, and "surrender" is not necessarily weak willed submission. Healthy control involves sensitivity to feedback, and a willingness to be flexible, creative and decisive. Healthy surrender involves letting go, trusting your environment and your relationships, and relaxing about your destiny.
>
> Control can exist in the midst of surrender, and surrender in the midst of control. Do you like to control things? Can you enjoy surrender? Do you fear the responsibility of control? In this session we explore with you the dance and the delicate balance of control and surrender.[19]

Dr. Rolf's Words Related to the Fourth Session

"On the floor of the pelvis, on its well-being and its organization is dependent the entire health of 1) the reproductive system, 2) the excretory system, and 3) the way in which the viscera will arrange themselves and support each other. As the floor gains support and balance, tone changes within the viscera, bringing new neurological and functional balance. Therefore the straightening of crooked legs takes on almost secondary importance in this hour."[20]

Practitioner Goals for the Fourth Session

✦ Align the midline of the legs.
✦ Release the pelvic floor.
✦ Get the legs to drop freely out of the pelvis.
✦ Get the patellae to float.
✦ Create sit bones that reach and adductors that span.

Areas Addressed

The areas addressed include the inner legs, hamstrings, pelvis, neck, and back. This is the first time that we anatomically address core structures along the inner line of the body that attach to the spine. Sessions one through three have helped establish balance in the front, back, and sides of the body. That previous work now allows the inner line to be addressed so everything can let go into it.

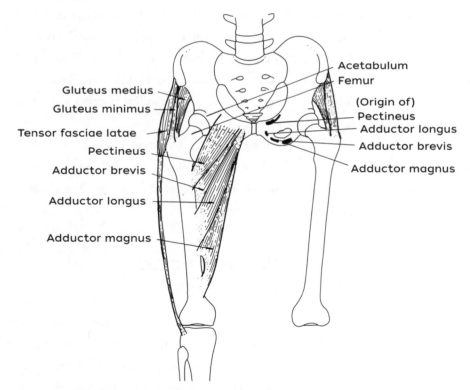

✦ Fig. 2.11. The adductor muscles of the inner thigh.

From *Rolfing: Reestablishing the Natural Alignment and Structural Integration of the Human Body for Vitality and Well-Being* by Ida P. Rolf, Ph.D. Reprinted with permission of publisher.

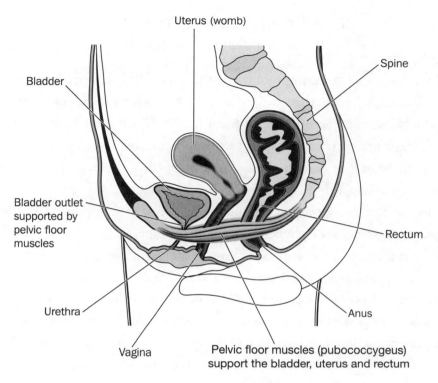

Uterus (womb)

Spine

Bladder

Bladder outlet
supported by
pelvic floor
muscles

Rectum

Urethra

Anus

Vagina

Pelvic floor muscles (pubococcygeus)
support the bladder, uterus and rectum

◆ Fig. 2.12. The pelvic floor.
From Blamb/Shutterstock.com

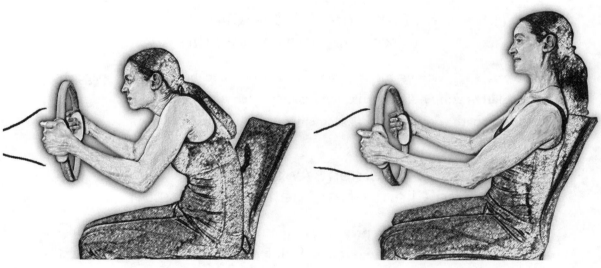

◆ Fig. 2.13. An "emotionally uptight" pelvic floor.

This illustration was produced by and used with kind
permission of Andreini McPherson-Husbands
and Andreina Shelton.

◆ Fig. 2.14. A relaxed pelvic floor.

This illustration was produced by and used with kind
permission of Andreini McPherson-Husbands
and Andreina Shelton.

The Energetics of the Line
in the Fourth Session

The fourth session marks the point where there is a shift in the energetic potential of the Rolf Line. I sense that the opportunity to work with the core-level pelvic floor can boost the practitioner and client into the quantum energetic aspect of the Rolfing work. Betsy Sise speaks to this in her book *The Rolfing Experience*. Sise says that Dr. Rolf described the similarity of the Earth and electromagnetic human body as having both an electric core and a magnetic sleeve. She contended that electric core energy would be able to flow freely through the body if blockages were removed on the physical and energetic levels.

Recently, one of my clients said to me at the beginning of his fourth session, "We are going to unstick the first chakra today." "Yes!" I exclaimed. He knew!

The first chakra is located at the base of the spine in the area of the pelvic floor. The floor of the pelvis may be strained by rotation patterns from the legs. In the fourth session, we begin to touch the energetics of this chakra. Issues regarding sexuality and survival may arise, particularly for people who have been sexually abused. The work of Structural Integration can be healing, and the fourth session is often a turning point.

Self-Care for the Client
after the Fourth Session

Follow the suggestions for self-care that are outlined beginning on page 39, particularly taking a short walk immediately after your session and taking your first detox bath within six hours. Remember to drink plenty of water.

Movement Awareness for
the Client after the Fourth Session

Tensions in the pelvic floor prevent us from truly relaxing. When we pull in at the pelvic floor and squeeze our anus tightly, our body will pull up and away from whatever is underneath us, be it the chair we are sitting on, the floor we stand on, or the bed we lie on. This tension does not allow for rest. The stress of a tight pelvic floor can be transmitted all the way up the spine to the head and neck. Such tensions activate the sympathetic fight-or-flight aspect of the autonomic nervous system.

Check on that now: Pull in at your pelvic floor and squeeze tightly at your anus. Follow the line of tension. It may extend all the way up your spine to your head and neck. Now take a big breath and let go there. Feel the letting down and letting go that happens. Feel the relaxation in your face. Notice how this letting go allows your body to rest completely and be supported by what is beneath it.

Karen's Story

In 2007, I worked with a woman who had been sexually abused. Three months after her tenth session, I interviewed Karen about her Structural Integration experience and made a transcript from the audio recording. The following excerpts are included with her permission.

Karen had been sexually abused when she was young. In the interview, she said, "I think what happened to me in that experience is I felt sexual arousal during something that intellectually made no sense to me and so I felt like my body was not my ally. My body was my enemy."

"Like you couldn't trust your body?" I asked.

"That's right."

"So there was perhaps a disassociation from your body?"

"Exactly," she said. "I think I felt that way for many, many years."

"Now," I said, "with the Structural Integration, there is a journey back into the body—really paying attention."

"And I think a lot of it had to do with watching you," she said.

"When you say watching me, what do you mean?"

"Well," said Karen, "I am a bodyworker. I am probably 50 pounds more than you in terms of body mass. I experience fatigue and drain, and I don't even do 75 percent of what you do in a session throughout my day! If I compare what I do in a day of work and what you do in a day of work, I might put out 25 percent of the amount of energy you do. I can remember you talking about how every time when you do a session, you drop in and you feel the Earth energy and you let that come through you. And I realized that I don't have that relationship."

"You didn't have that connection," I stated.

"That's right," she said.

"Did it make sense as I started talking about it?"

"It made a lot of sense. It started making sense as I watched your body and the strength you have as you go through a whole session and you don't feel fatigued or drained. I know it's not self-generated energy. You're allowing energy to come *through* you. And I think that there's no way for that to happen if you feel like your body is something that you can't trust. How can you let any of that energy work through you? Does that make sense?"

"Yes," I said. "There is such truth in your words."

"During my fourth session," said Karen, "I noticed pelvic floor holding, clenching, the feeling of needing to keep it all together. I experienced both sadness and understanding in my body tissues of where it all began."

"I remember that session with you," I said. "Somehow I could feel that your body was pulling up off the table, and I said, 'Karen, just let it down. Let the table support you.' I felt like you hadn't truly rested for years. You hadn't let down to be supported."

"It took me until the fourth session to trust you to do that," said Karen. "I had enough experience in the first three sessions to know there was a difference between pain of tissue damage and the pain of releasing stuck pain.

"I can remember when you were working around my pelvic floor," she continued. "I felt the holding I was talking about and felt sad about being out of balance with that energy within myself. How much energy I used and wasted, holding it all together, when there is something there that was made to hold it together for me. If you don't have a good relationship with your original mother and father, how can you have a good relationship with those two energies?"

In reflecting on her eighth session (a lower body session), Karen read to me some thoughts she had written: "If we trust and surrender and rest into the soles of our feet, the Earth energy will rise up into and through us. And the heavens will fall down and into us. We become the sacred space of their sacred marriage in connection between Mother Earth and Father Sky. Our potential is infinite. If we are unable to surrender and allow, we are left to stand on our own volition. The energy of the Earth and heavens has no place within us to meet and create love in and through us. We begin to age and cripple because we are not living our purpose in life. Our purpose in life is to be the connection between that marriage."

After reading that to me, Karen looked up and said, "But then again, with the kind of relationship that I had with my mother and father, how could I even trust to let that energy happen?"

"That was then, and this is now," I said. "You were able to make that jump to choose something different. You started to feel it."

"Yes," said Karen. "The neat thing is, we can have that mother/father relationship outside of the one we had as a kid. For so many of us, when we had that relationship, it was really dysfunctional."

The work that Karen and I did together helped her clear blockages in her body, mind, and emotions. It helped her reframe her experience and choose something different. It helped her evolve in her body, mind, emotion, and spirit. That is the potential within Structural Integration!

Between the Fourth and Fifth Sessions

Beginning with session four, we enter the core-level work of Structural Integration—the deep sessions. Old feelings and emotions often surface during sessions four, five, six, and seven. In the fourth session, we enter the core of the body from the inside line of the legs and the floor of the pelvis. This session begins to establish the Line through the center of the torso along the front of the spine by balancing the inside of the legs and the pelvic floor. This work can stir up emotional holding patterns.

With the fourth session, we have begun to touch the core of the body and mind. Emotions that have been locked in the pelvis and legs may become stirred. Joseph Heller described this as an opportunity to think about the areas in your life where you like to control and dominate, as compared to the areas in which you are more surrendered. During those moments when you like to control things, see if you can consciously relax your pelvic floor. Does that change your experience?

Work in the fourth session addresses muscles that pull down on the pelvis. Note that sometimes symptoms appear to worsen at this time because we have begun to open up the core of the body. Some people feel an energetic division after this session because we are only opening up the lower half of the front line of the body. The following sessions will help bring integration and balance to your body. You will do best *not to make any major life changes between sessions four and five*. And be sure to receive your fifth session in a timely manner, as it will help balance your body.

As we've noted, the Structural Integration process will have its ups and downs while the body is being balanced and cleared of strain. It is important to be gentle with yourself, especially during these deep core-level sessions. Cut yourself slack. Ask others to do the same. "The pot is being stirred right now," so to speak. Patience and gentleness with yourself are essential during this time of clearing.

Regarding stress and its effects on the body, Dr. Rolf said:

Serious traumatic episodes leave their mark and are anchored literally in the flesh of the body. Until the flesh of the body is freed so that it can move appropriately to the pattern, the traumatic episode cannot really be erased or forgotten from that body. It is not possible. . . .

Personality expresses a two-sided coin. One side is the physical, and one side is the mental. A serious change in either one will most seriously result in serious change in the other.[22]

SESSION FIVE
The Guts

The Theme of the Fifth Session

Joseph Heller described the theme of the fifth session as "the guts." He said:

> The function of the guts—stomach, intestines, and other abdominal organs—is to process energy, particularly in the form of food. Our relationship with food is a great metaphor for our relationship with love and nurturance. Do you tend to metabolize and eliminate very rapidly, so that you eliminate and push away any possible excess food—or love? Do you tend to retain food—or do you hold on to the signs or forms of love—perhaps feeling there is a scarcity of sustenance whether in the form of food or love? The guts are also the place where we feel our strongest feelings or emotions, our "gut feelings." What gut feelings do you most often feel? Are there any that you suppress or avoid? Finally, the guts are associated with courage and strength of character. Do you have guts? When do you—when don't you?[23]

Dr. Rolf's Words Related to the Fifth Session

"If a body is normal, the psoas should elongate during flexion and fall back toward the spine. . . . By virtue of this, the normal psoas forms an important part of a supporting web holding the lumbar vertebrae appropriately spanned."[24]

"Structural weakness or metabolic insufficiency in the psoas thereby inevitably affects the lumbar plexus and its autonomic neighbors. If the psoas is inadequate, local nutritional exchange is disturbed, as is the metabolic rate in the lower digestive tract (specifically basic elimination as well as food absorption)."[25]

Practitioner Goals
for the Fifth Session

✦ Lengthen the front of the body's core so the pelvis becomes more horizontal.

✦ Balance and release the deep muscles of the pelvis.

✦ Achieve rectus abdominis/psoas balance.

Areas Addressed

This session is about lengthening the core muscles in the front of the torso. It is a deep session. Your practitioner may begin the session by releasing the more superficial muscles of the quadriceps at the top of the legs in the front of the body. Next, the rectus abdominis, a superficial muscle that extends from the pubic bone to the rib cage, is released. Work may be needed in the ribs in the front and back of the chest in order to help the rectus abdominis lengthen. The shoulder girdle in the arms and shoulders may be addressed as well.

Then your practitioner will work to lengthen and balance the deeper core muscles of the psoas and iliacus, assisting the pelvis in becoming more horizontal, which is a major goal of *every* session of Structural Integration. The pelvis can easily be horizontal with the psoas being back against the spine. It is important to breathe during this work to help your tissues release. Let each exhalation help your body relax into the table.

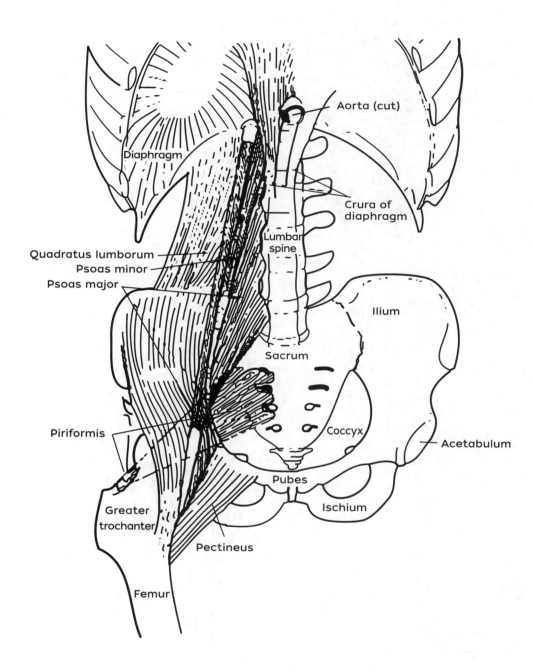

✦ Fig. 2.15. The muscles of the abdomen.

From *Rolfing: Reestablishing the Natural Alignment and Structural Integration of the Human Body for Vitality and Well-Being* by Ida P. Rolf, Ph.D. Reprinted with permission of publisher.

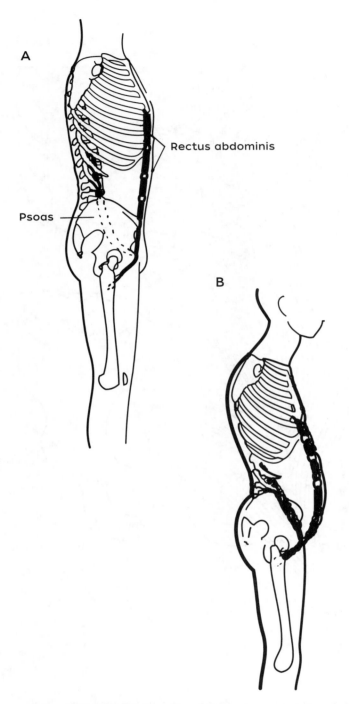

✦ Fig. 2.16. The relationship of the psoas and rectus abdominis:
(A) balanced psoas; (B) short, contracted psoas.

From *Rolfing: Reestablishing the Natural Alignment and Structural Integration of the Human Body for Vitality and Well-Being* by Ida P. Rolf, Ph.D. Reprinted with permission of publisher.

The Energetics of the
Line in the Fifth Session

Humans have an inherent connection into fields of energy that are greater than our own. I call these greater energy fields "Source energy."

Source energy includes the energy of the heavens and the Earth. It is the electromagnetic life force that is derived from gravitational fields. It runs through our bodies and supports, nourishes, and energizes us. All life is sustained by it. Embedded within its fields of energy is information. The source of that energy is Love.

When our body segments are aligned and gravity flows through, we can connect into these higher energy fields that support us and move through us. We can let go of "efforting" as individuals and partner up with that universal energy. We don't have to go it alone. It's about being "in the flow," as the Taoists would say. Structural Integration can enhance that connection. It *can* be experienced. *You* can experience it.

I remember working with a young woman in Hawaii whose pelvis was very anterior. We had done a lot of work to lengthen the associated structures, but when she stood up, her hips went right back into their accustomed anterior position. So I placed one of my hands on the front of her lower abdomen and the other on the back of her sacrum. While being silently present with her, I asked myself what was still contributing to her old pattern. In that moment of inner reflection, it became clear to me that efforting seemed to be a significant part of her anterior pelvis. Efforting arises out of the belief that we have to struggle to make things happen. So I initiated a conversation with her about that belief.

Then I helped position her pelvis into a neutral alignment. Because of the work we had done, her body had the potential to go there, but she had no experience of that position. As I gently pressed her sacrum down, her anterior pelvis lifted. We both had a moment of appreciation as she found her core from the inside and lengthened from the bottom of her feet to the top of her head through her inner Line.

Her horizontal pelvis now offered her the opportunity to explore and connect into those larger fields of supportive energy. When the pelvis is anterior, the flow of life force is blocked. The subtle energy of the Earth cannot flow all the way up, and the energy coming through the top has difficulty moving down.

Please note: If I had not been able to guide her to experience that "aha" moment, her session would not have been as complete or effective. A client's conscious awareness helps maximize the integration of their physical changes.

As we have discussed, when the energies from above and below meet in the center of the body, a union of the yin and yang, of the positive and negative poles of the body, occurs. A joining together or marriage takes place between those energies. That energy is then spun by the chakras into the meridian system that lies within the connective tissues of the body and then out into the energy field surrounding the body. "In sessions four and five," said Emmett, "an inside Line has been created that is continuous all the way to the neck. In the fifth session, a series of centers have been activated through the chakras."

If we can align ourselves with larger fields of energy, we don't have to work so hard. When I get on my Line, I breathe and invite those energies into my body, and I feel tingling sensations move through me. When I do that consciously, I open up to those energies, and sometimes information moves through me like a download. Life becomes easier.

⚘ Exercise: Feeding Your Body with Energy

Feel your fifth-session Line now. Notice your feet. Let your body weight fall in front of your ankles. Your feet are ear width apart. Feel where the top of your head is. Your hips drop like weights from the end of your spine. Your shoulders are resting on and supported by your ribs below them. Neither pulled forward nor back, they rest like a coat hanger over your ribs. Keep your knees soft with give, not locked. Locked knees may cause the hips to tilt forward.

Keep your line of vision parallel to the floor. Women all around the world and people who carry negative emotions look downward as a matter of training and habit. A level gaze is essential to empowerment, as well as proper alignment.

Now breathe from your feet to the top of your head. Then let your breath move from the top of your head down to your feet. Open your feet and head to the subtle electromagnetic energies of the heavens above and the Earth below. Invite that energy into your body. It is food for every cell. Your breath is the pump that moves that energy. Use your breath to draw that energy into your body. Can you feel the tingling sensations move up your legs from your feet and down into your body from the top of your head? That is life force lighting you up!

Self-Care for the Client
after the Fifth Session

Follow the suggestions for self-care that are outlined beginning on page 39, particularly taking a short walk immediately after your session and taking your first detox bath within six hours. Remember to drink plenty of water.

Movement Awareness for the Client
after the Fifth Session

"Tuck your hips under. Suck your belly in. Stand up straight, and throw your shoulders back. Pretend you have a dollar bill rolled up between your butt cheeks, and squeeze it so tight that it won't fall out! Now press that coin you're holding between your knees so tightly that it won't fall out either." Does any of that sound familiar? These are postural cues that some of us grew up with. Maybe you have a few of your own. We have been given postural cues that are *counterproductive* all of our lives.

Holding the body in any of these forced unnatural postures creates strain in the viscera and holding patterns that will extend through the connective tissues from one end of the body to the other. That strain can also activate nerves that are part of the fight-or-flight sympathetic branch of the autonomic nervous system. It's no wonder people have bought into concepts like "buns of steel" and "abs of steel." We were taught to accept those ideas as children. But really! How comfortable are those bodies to actually live in?

I created similar strain patterns in my body with my gymnastics training as a child. I can still hear my coach say, "Squeeze your butt as tight as a pencil." That's how I could fly through the air with the greatest of ease. Done enough times, the body remembers, and remembers. Through repetition, tight connective tissues can set up long-term strain patterns in the body.

In gymnastics training, we did a lot of abdominal conditioning, including sit-ups, crunches, and leg lifts. Done improperly, the rectus abdominis (a superficial belly muscle) pulls forward along with the psoas beneath it. And because the psoas muscles are attached to the spine, the spine pulls forward as well. This creates an excessive arch in the lower back known as lordosis. It also contributes to a protruding belly because the abdominal contents will spill forward as a result of the forward rotation of the pelvis. When this happens, the psoas muscles shorten and the abdominal muscles get overstretched and stuck in that position.

Doing sit-ups can help firm up the rectus abdominis and help a little with the potbelly, but it's temporary. Emmett said, "You can't keep doing more and more sit-ups. Eventually it could lead to kyphosis," a rounding of the upper back due to a shortening in the midsection. What is needed is a horizontal pelvis. And that comes by lengthening the psoas muscles and balancing the rectus abdominis. Joseph Heller said, "A long lean look comes from lengthening the psoas, not from shortening the rectus abdominis."[26] An excessive number of sit-ups also can create problems with constipation. The viscera below those tight abs can get so tied up in knots that things just will not move through!

Many of us are trying to have good posture. That is a commendable goal. But forcing good posture can create problems.

The focus in Structural Integration is to organize and balance the center of gravity of the major body segments. This allows gravity to flow through so that it can become a beneficial force and standing, sitting, and walking can happen with ease. Forced abnormal posture in a body filled with patterns of strain creates fatigue and cannot be sustained for very long. It goes "against the flow."

Between the Fifth and Sixth Sessions

Between sessions five and six, Joseph Heller suggested that people pay attention to their guts. He said, "Be aware of your emotions and how they relate to tension in your body, particularly in your guts. As emotions come up, breathe into your guts and feel your emotions as fully as you can. How does this feel? What happens in your body?"[27]

This is the time to recommit to your Structural Integration series. Sessions four through seven are the core-level sessions. Your body will need them to balance. Emmett said, "If a person has to quit the series, quitting after five is better than after four. The seventh hour is an even better place to quit because the electrical body and autonomic system have been tuned by then."

SESSION SIX
Holding Back

The Theme of the Sixth Session

Joseph Heller tells us:

> The theme of this session is "Holding Back," which literally describes tension or holding in one's back, and figuratively describes the ways we limit our self-expression, power and creativity. These limits are physically embodied as tension in the extensor muscles along the spine. In the process of growing up, most of us develop patterns of holding back that may seem necessary, such as not speaking or moving during school or not fully expressing our excitement or sadness. Now these same patterns, chronically ingrained in our character, limit our expression of love, power, and creativity. What expression or emotion do you hold back? How do you hold back your power? As the tension in your back releases, whatever has been held back—love, anger, joy, sadness— can begin to emerge, giving you a new opportunity to express and communicate more freely.[28]

Dr. Rolf's Words Related to the Sixth Session

"If stress is to be relieved, it is important that no myofascial component contributing to pelvic balance be overlooked . . . other muscle groups also participate in pelvic movement—hamstrings, the gluteal group (maximus, medius, and minimus), and the so-called rotators underlying the gluteus maximus."[29]

Practitioner Goals for
the Sixth Session

+ Lengthen the back of the body's core from the heels to the neck.
+ Balance and lengthen the muscles that surround and support
   the spine.
+ Release and lengthen the deep muscles of the buttocks,
   pelvis, and legs.

Areas Addressed

This session is about lengthening the core of the back of the body to match the work of session five on the front of the body. Most of this session is done with the client lying on his or her stomach. Areas addressed include the legs, hips, back, and neck. The practitioner will also work to ease the muscles deep in the hips known as the rotators, the hamstrings, and the calf muscles, as well as the muscles along the length of the spine called the erector spinae.

The sixth session is sometimes called the hour of the breathing pelvis because it has the capacity to wake the sacrum, the triangularly shaped bone in the pelvis at the base of the spine. A free pelvis rocks forward with respiration. When you get the sacrum breathing, you have a core that is alive. The hallmark of a good sixth session is when the spine lengthens as it breathes and the client's breath is reflected in his or her entire rib cage, spine, and pelvis.

The Energetics of
the Line in the Sixth Session

Rotations in the body have a way of shortening and compressing the width and length of the joints. After a sixth session, people will often look and feel taller because of the length gained through work in the legs, along the spinal column, and in the hips. Not only does the physical body lengthen, but the energetic field of the body will also expand.

Rosemary Feitis, D.O., and R. Louis Schultz, Ph.D., advanced certified Rolfer, Rolfing Movement teacher, and founder of the anatomy program at the Rolf Institute, examined connective tissues and the loosening of tight fascial

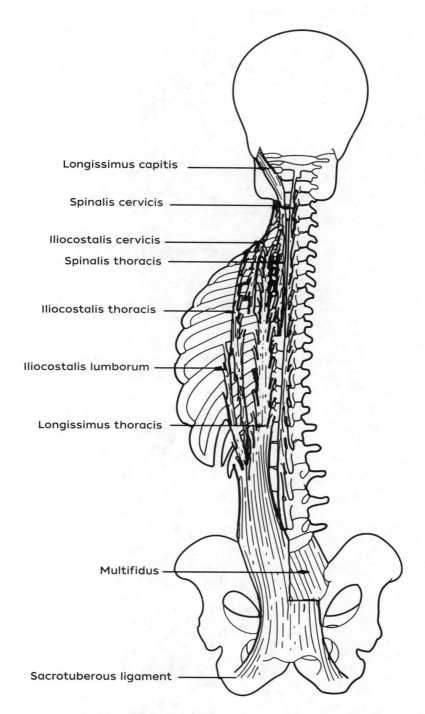

Longissimus capitis

Spinalis cervicis

Iliocostalis cervicis

Spinalis thoracis

Iliocostalis thoracis

Iliocostalis lumborum

Longissimus thoracis

Multifidus

Sacrotuberous ligament

◆ Fig. 2.17. The spine and the erector spinae muscles.

From *Rolfing: Reestablishing the Natural Alignment and Structural Integration of the Human Body for Vitality and Well-Being* by Ida P. Rolf, Ph.D. Reprinted with permission of publisher.

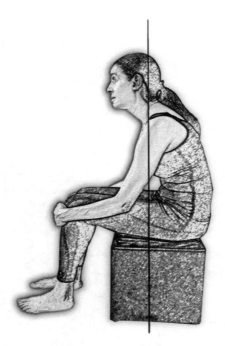

✦ Fig. 2.18. Imbalanced pelvic base.

This illustration was produced by and used with kind permission of
Andreini McPherson-Husbands and Andreina Shelton.

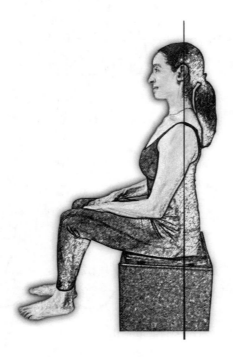

✦ Fig. 2.19. Balanced pelvic base.

This illustration was produced by and used with kind permission of
Andreini McPherson-Husbands and Andreina Shelton.

bands in the body in order to create greater length, energy, and freedom of movement in their article "A Rolfian Review of Anatomy." They stated, "What we have presented is an anatomical description of a body language. Whether it is interpreted in term(s) of emotional blocks, energy centers, or structural bandings, the goal remains the same. When the soft tissue releases, the joints are able to 'float,' increasing awareness and mobility in the body. Such responses must lead to lifting upward while remaining grounded—Ida Rolf's vision of verticality in relation to gravity."[30]

During a training in Kauai in 2012 my teacher Emmett shared some interesting insights about the Line. He said:

We are trying to get a Line all the way through to the bottom of the feet. I have spent forty years trying to get my weight down into the ground, because if you can get your weight completely down into the ground, then you will weigh nothing! There is nothing to lift! You are totally supported by the gravitational field. The whole idea is how to get your weight down, not how to get up! Up is automatic. Up happens all by itself. Down doesn't. Whatever goes down must come up, which is the opposite of what you learn in your physics class.

If the body segments are stacked properly, the body has no weight and it doesn't take anything to keep it there. And if you are open in the field that you're stacked in and you move in such a way that you don't lose that, you keep balanced in the field. You don't weigh anything because the weight is all going down. Ida thought that we would never have to sleep a wink at night if we literally swam in the energy field that is available to us all the time!

The Line does come through the center of the cylinder of both legs. We want to get the legs to become open channels into the Earth. Ida's whole idea, metaphysically, was that the calcaneus, the heel, should act like a root chakra in classic literature. The heel should be grounded into the Earth as the root chakra is for meditating. So it's the ability of the legs to feel alive. The width of the feet while standing are about the same as the width of the ears. Very few people get their feet down in the same direction. One foot will usually be internally rotated while the other foot is externally rotated.[31]

Dr. Rolf said that if you are stuck in your evolution, if you are stuck in your growth, if you are not getting any better, if you are not getting any more connected to the ground, if your aches and pains are continuing and you can't get out of it, the answer to your problems will always partly be in the legs. That's where your evolution gets stuck: from the legs.

⚘ Exercise: Weighting Down

As you stand after your sixth session, find your Line. Let your weight drop down in front of your ankles. Let your hips drop like a weight from the end of your spine. Your knees are soft with give. Let yourself be supported by the surface you are standing on.

To activate the center of your Line, take a breath and then exhale, pressing your diaphragm fully down at the end of your exhalation. Engage your diaphragm in this way as you continue to breathe. Activating your diaphragm will optimize your structural alignment by activating core-level muscles in the abdominal area, drawing back the lumbar and cervical vertebrae at each end of the spine.

Notice how grounded and rooted your feet suddenly become as you activate your core in this way. Feel your weight drop down into the floor or Earth. Become aware, as well, of the *up* spot at the top of your head.

Sense the lightness and quality of lift that runs through the center of your being along the front side of your spine. From your waist down, your body weight can drop down into the floor or Earth that is supporting you. From your waist up, there is a possibility of effortless lift along the front side of your spine up through the top of your head. In the middle of your body, your core-level muscles are engaged, supporting the length of your spine from one end to the other.

Breathe from the bottom of your feet to the top of your head, letting your breath move and expand with ease. Bring a breath in from the top of your head and send it down your central Line to the bottom of your feet. You have become the conduit, connecting your energy field with that of the Earth and cosmos, from one end of your body to the other.

Self-Care for the Client
after the Sixth Session

Follow the suggestions for self-care that are outlined beginning on page 39, particularly taking a short walk immediately after your session and taking your first detox bath within six hours. Remember to drink plenty of water.

Be sure to find some time to get your bare feet on the Earth, naturally reducing inflammation as you ground, and practice feeling your weight drop down.

A Himalayan salt sole (pronounced "solay"), a weak brine of naturally mineral-rich salt, can be particularly useful now to help reduce calcification in tissues and joints. See page 131 for directions for making it.

Movement Awareness for the Client
after the Sixth Session

During sessions four through seven, your practitioner is helping to activate small muscles in the core of your body next to the spine. These are known as the *intrinsic* muscles. You can focus your attention on using these small core-level muscles in an undulation exercise.

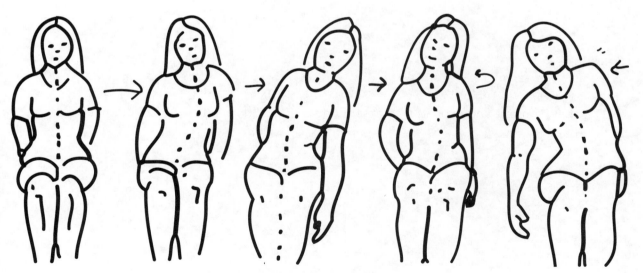

✦ Fig. 2.20. Undulation moving from psoas.
This drawing was adapted by Carolyn Cameron from the Hellerwork *Client's Handbook*
and used with kind permission of Hellerwork International, LLC.

⚸ Exercise: Undulation

Sit in a chair and let your spine sway from side to side. Let the movement originate at your spine and flow outward to the rest of your body. You can use the image of being pulled from side to side by a string attached to the center of your chest. How does this feel? You can also undulate from front to back.[32]

Undulating movements help keep your spine flexible and long. Our bodies may have forgotten how to undulate, but we can bring articulation back with some practice.

Between the Sixth and Seventh Sessions

Your head and neck may feel uncomfortable after the sixth session. A lot of order has been established from the ankles upward in the core structure. The least symmetry is now in the cranium and the neck.

In the seventh session, the head and neck will be balanced on top of the Line that has been established in the previous sessions. At this point in the series, a client may experience some psychological vulnerability. It is best not to have a large gap of time between sessions six and seven.

SESSION SEVEN
Losing Your Head

The Theme
of the Seventh Session

Joseph Heller described the theme of this session as "losing your head." He said:

> By that we mean releasing excessive attention to the analytic, mental, and inward processes that apparently occur in the head. Our culture tends to emphasize these processes at the expense of body awareness with the result that many people experience their body as only a vehicle to transport the all-important head. The mind and the ability to think are certainly great assets. It is only when we use our rational processes to the exclusion of our other capacities that we become limited in our feeling and intuition. Do you like to have rational answers for everything? How do you balance using your feelings and thought processes to guide you in life? This session returns you to a more balanced relationship between head and body, and between reason and feeling.[33]

Dr. Rolf's Words Related to
the Seventh Session

"For balance, the neck structure must be spaced midway with respect to the sides of the body, and seem midway with respect to the front and back. Alignment, a satisfying balance, requires that only a vertical cervical spine can form the upper segment of a vertically stacked body."[34]

Practitioner Goals
for the Seventh Session

✦ Release and lengthen the top of the core.

✦ Align and balance the head, neck, and shoulder girdle over the torso.

✦ Restore freedom of movement to the head and jaw.

✦ Release tension in the head, face, and neck.

✦ Restore symmetry and freedom of expression to the face.

Areas Addressed

At this point in the series, the major body segments of the torso have become more aligned along a central core. This session is about balancing the head and neck on top of that core line. Joseph Heller said, "In an unaligned body, the neck commonly leans forward, the head tilts backward, [and] the muscles of the neck become filled with tension. In a balanced body, the neck is a vertical pillar sitting on top of the horizontal surface of the shoulder girdle. The head rests on the top of the neck, without needing constant tension in the back of the neck to hold it on. This balanced position allows effortless motion of the head and jaw."[35] The head, neck, and "yoke" of the shoulder girdle can now align over the frame of the body without effort or strain. This session includes work to release strained musculature in the face, which allows for freedom of full facial expression. It also facilitates a more balanced relationship between reason and feeling as excessive tension is released in the head, face, and neck.

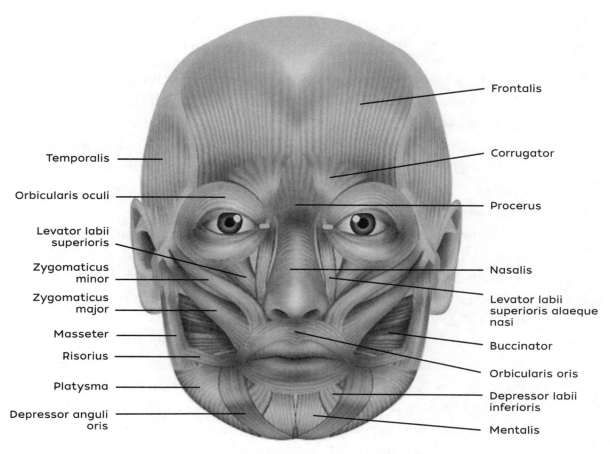

Frontalis

Corrugator

Temporalis

Orbicularis oculi

Procerus

Levator labii
superioris

Zygomaticus
minor

Nasalis

Zygomaticus
major

Levator labii
superioris alaeque
nasi

Masseter

Buccinator

Risorius

Orbicularis oris

Platysma

Depressor labii
inferioris

Depressor anguli
oris

Mentalis

✦ Fig. 2.21. The muscles of the face.
From Tefi/Shutterstock.com

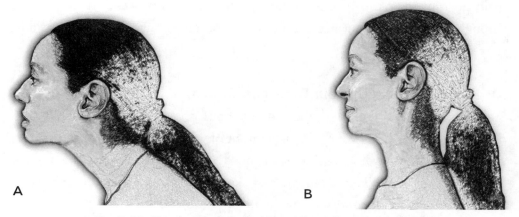

A

B

✦ Fig. 2.22. Head and neck position: (A) unaligned; (B) aligned.
These illustrations were produced by and used with kind permission of
Andreini McPherson-Husbands and Andreina Shelton.

The Energetics of the Line
in the Seventh Session

"How did you become so aware of this Line in your body?" a client asked me.

I've experienced subtle flows of life-force energy in my body for years, but I didn't know what they were doing for me. Now we have the science that proves their health benefits. It's like tapping into a source of free energy. The energy is out there. It's available to us. We swim in a sea of energy. It's just a matter of how we can maximize its flow through the body. And being on my Line is one of the best ways I know to do that.

With the seventh session, it becomes possible to have a more complete experience of this Line in our body. A true connection with the larger fields of energy that surround us is now available from head to toe. We can more deeply and consciously connect with the electromagnetic life-force energy that runs through both ends of the central axis of our body along our Line.

Emmett said that the sixth and seventh sessions are considered to be electrical tune-ups for the body. The negative pole is at the heels, and the positive pole is in the brain stem. "Upright primates are the only animals that have a bioelectrical system," said Emmett. "Other animals are on magnetic lines. The magnetic lines of force run in horizontals around the Earth. Electrical lines run in ninety-degree planes. When we get our electrical lines clean through Structural Integration, our bioelectrical systems become more efficient."

By the end of your seventh session, your neck and head will be more optimally positioned on top of your shoulder girdle. The ability of the breath to move through the center of your neck and head has become enhanced as evidenced in the following exercise.

⅋ Exercise: Tuning Up Your Bioelectric System

Stand now with your feet well supported by the Earth. Let all of your weight drop down into the center of your feet just in front of your ankles. Above your ankles, your body becomes weightless. Let your knees be soft. Your hips drop like weights from your spine, and your shoulders rest like a coat hanger over your rib cage. Feel and know where the top of your head—your *up*—is.

Take a breath, and imagine with that breath that you are drawing universal life force into your body from the surface of the Earth. Feel it move into your feet, up the central line of your body in front of the spine, and out through the top of your head into the energy field that surrounds you. *Notice how your head gently bobbles backward in relation to the movement of your ribs and breath.* Each gentle backward bobble of your head helps align the head and neck into a more balanced position on top of your shoulder girdle. Allow your breath to move directly out of the top of your head as you draw the breath up from your feet with your inhale. See if you can also move the energy in the other direction by drawing it in through the top of your head with an inhale, and then send it down into your body with your exhale.

As you continue to breathe, feel your breath working like a pump, drawing energy from the top of your head downward and from your feet upward. You may notice subtle tingling sensations moving through you. In this moment, your body has become a conduit of energetic connection between the life-force energy of the larger electromagnetic fields of the Earth and heavens. Every cell, tissue, and major organ system in your body can be supported by it. Fill your body with this energy. Allow length to arise from within yourself as you experience this sensation of being on your Line.

Self-Care for the Client after the Seventh Session

Immediately after the seventh session, I recommend that my clients chill. I often have clients lie on the mat of my BEMER, an electromagnetic healing device that pulses a gentle electromagnetic energy. It's a great way to integrate the work of a Structural Integration session before shifting back into the activities of the day.

Also follow the suggestions for self-care that are outlined beginning on page 39, particularly taking a short walk immediately after your session and taking your first detox bath within six hours. Remember to drink plenty of water.

Movement Awareness for the Client after the Seventh Session

Notice the position of your head over your shoulders. Perhaps you can feel more lift ease and length through your Line now. Cultivate that awareness. Optimal vertical alignment of the head over the shoulder girdle supports balanced alignment in the rest of the body.

From the Hellerwork perspective on movement awareness, because the seventh session addresses areas of strain in the head and neck, it allows full range of movement in our facial muscles, which allow us to reveal emotion. Are you able to express a full range of emotions through your facial movements? Do your facial expressions adequately reflect your feelings, or do you feel like you are wearing a mask?

How you carry your head during movement is important. When you are reaching down to pick something up, release strain in the back of your neck by letting your head go instead of holding your head up. When you are walking, imagine that your head is moving freely and easily on top of a spring. Notice how relaxed and loose that can feel.[36]

Between the Seventh and Eighth Sessions

Due to the work done in the previous core sessions, deeper layers of strain may now be surfacing in your lower body. If this is the case for you, take heart! These deeper layers of strain that are now finally surfacing are ready to be released. And that is a good thing! Your practitioner will address these patterns of strain in session eight.

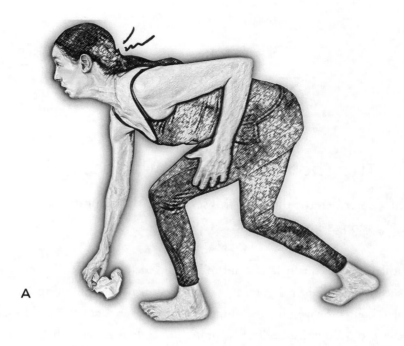

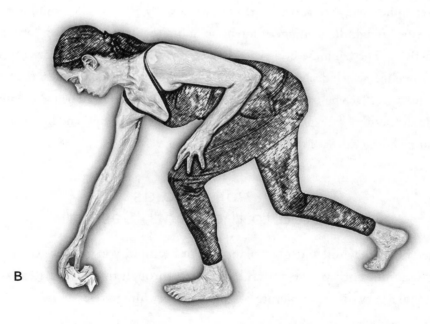

✦ Fig. 2.23. (A) Neck holding while bending; (B) head released while bending.

These illustrations were produced by and used with kind permission of
Andreini McPherson-Husbands and Andreina Shelton.

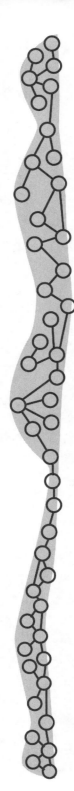

SESSION EIGHT
The Feminine

The Theme of the Eighth Session

Joseph Heller described the theme of this session as "the feminine" and the theme of the ninth session as "the masculine." He noted:

> Both principles are equally important in life, and each exists within every person, male or female. The pelvic girdle and legs represent the feminine principle. The pelvis houses the womb—the ultimate symbol of nurturance—and the legs connect us to Mother Earth. The feminine principle represents the power of attraction. Where masculine energy works through action and directed effort, feminine energy radiates and draws in whatever is desired. The feminine manifests through the medium of intention and receptivity, rather than form and activity. The feminine deals with beauty and well-being, complementing the masculine, which deals with order and the law. How do you manifest the feminine style? Do you trust this approach to life and the power of being receptive? In this session, we explore how you use the feminine principle and how you can bring it into balance in your life.[37]

Dr. Rolf's Words
Related to the Eighth Session

"The body as a whole must be balanced. For example, you cannot get movement into a sacrum until you've gotten balance up through the thorax. Realizing this gives you a very different picture of how a totality integrates."[38]

Practitioner Goals
for the Eighth Session

✦ Release rotations in the lower half of the body.
✦ Balance the superficial and deep muscles of the legs, hips, and pelvis.
✦ To organize the lower girdle and connect into the lumbodorsal hinge.

Areas Addressed

The lower body is the focus of this session. Areas addressed include the feet, ankles, knees, and legs, which support the pelvis. Heller compared the pelvis to a bowl that holds the abdominal contents. In this session, core-level strain in the lower body often emerges to the surface of the body from the deeper work that has been done in sessions four through seven. I call this phenomenon the "causative strain." This deeper strain that may have been part of the original problem now becomes available to be addressed at the surface of the body. As that strain is released, an even tone of ease can spread through the musculature and layers of connective tissue.

Joseph Heller said, "Structurally, the purpose of this session is to balance the rotations in the lower half of the body." He compared the effect of rotation in the body to a twisted towel that shortens with rotation. In the same way, rotation in a leg can shorten it, which then imbalances the pelvis. This in turn creates an uneven base of support for the upper body that can affect the entire body.[39]

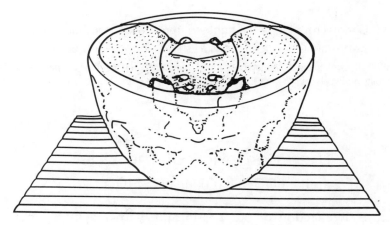

✦ Fig. 2.24. The pelvic bowl.

From *Rolfing: Reestablishing the Natural Alignment and Structural Integration of the Human Body for Vitality and Well-Being* by Ida P. Rolf, Ph.D. Reprinted with permission of publisher.

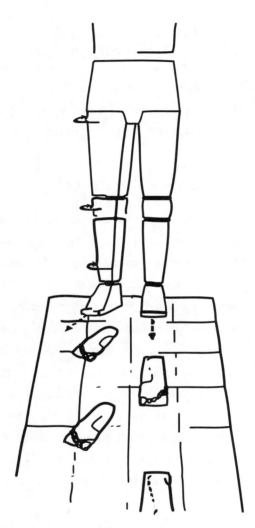

✦ Fig. 2.25. External rotation in the right leg makes it shorter than the left leg and creates an imbalanced pelvis as shown in these footprints.

From *Rolfing: Reestablishing the Natural Alignment and Structural Integration of the Human Body for Vitality and Well-Being* by Ida P. Rolf, Ph.D. Reprinted with permission of publisher.

The Energetics of the Line in the Eighth Session

Our posture is a reflection of our relationship with gravity. As our posture changes, so too does our relationship with gravity. As the body segments align and balance, energy from the electromagnetic fields of the heavens and Earth flows through us and supports us. We become living conduits as those streaming energies course through our body with our movements, feelings, and breath. Our mind and body begin to resonate with a sense of wholeness and connection. Confidence rises.

Because of the inseparable connection between body, mind, emotion, and spirit, as our posture changes, we can experience profound physiological and psychological shifts as well.

In the eighth-session Line, the lower body is connected into the lumbar spine at our core, and now movement can be initiated from the center of the body. As a balanced vertical Line meets a balanced horizontal line of the pelvic girdle, the physical and mental bodies become more congruent and integrated. And with the connection of the body to larger fields of energy through the Line, we experience more consistent energy and focus to help sustain our intentions. Our goals are more readily actualized in the world. The natural mental and emotional awakening of an integrated body literally supports the transformation of our becoming all we can be. Feel your Line now. Breathe fully and enjoy!

Self-Care for the Client after the Eighth Session

This session is about connecting the lower body into the core of the body and then initiating movement from the core. Follow the suggestions for self-care that are outlined beginning on page 39, particularly taking a short walk immediately after your session and taking your first detox bath within six hours. Remember to drink plenty of water. While taking a walk after your session, notice how fluid your walking movement can be as you move from the center of your body.

Movement Awareness for the Client after the Eighth Session

This session is about connecting the lower part of the body with the core or center of the body and then moving from that place of connectedness with the center.

⚘ Exercise: Moving from Your Center

Imagine that your body is a five-pointed star. Your arms, legs, and head are the points of the star, and your core or center is the middle of it. What is the feeling in the center of your body? Does energy move from the center of your body out through your extremities, or does it feel stuck in the middle?

Think of your body as having an upper half and a lower half. Which half draws most of your attention? Do you feel a connection between both halves of your body? Can one half of your body provide connection and support to the other? Create some communication or connection between the two halves.

Engage in a movement where your legs and pelvis are working, like running, hiking, or swimming. Do the activity with the movement originating from the core of your body, letting your core lengthen as you relax your pelvic floor. Now do the movement as if it were originating from the sleeve or outer wrap of the body. What differences do you notice? Did your movement feel more fluid when it originated from the core of your body?

Notice how far your breath moves when you inhale. Does it move all the way to the top of your head? Can it move to the bottom of your feet?

Review the exercises for finding the standing Line (page 37) and finding the sitting Line (page 38). At this point in your series, the core level alignment of your physical structure has been tuned up, allowing you to move even more life-force energy through your body. Become aware of the movement of this qi through the core of your body, extending along your Line through the center of your pelvic and shoulder girdles, connecting you to these larger fields of energy.

Between the Eighth and Ninth Sessions

Between the eighth and ninth sessions, you may notice deeper strain that has surfaced in your upper body. That is the recipe at work. Your practitioner will address those areas in the ninth session.

From the Hellerwork perspective, "consider the role of the feminine principle in your life. Notice an area of your life where hard work is not getting results. This could be at work, in relationships, or in creative activities. Relax your effort, while maintaining your attention and intention on your desired results. Assume they will come to you. See what happens."[40]

SESSION NINE
The Masculine

The Theme of the Ninth Session

Joseph Heller described the theme of this session as "the masculine." He noted:

> The arms, shoulder girdle and chest embody the masculine principle: doing, accomplishing, achieving. The masculine principle is the path of initiation, penetrating force, insight, and action. The masculine represents activity with purpose and movement with direction. Western culture emphasizes the masculine style, perhaps to the point of imbalance. Many people strain to work hard: "no pain—no gain." Even people with jobs that are not physically strenuous have tension throughout their bodies as a result of this attitude of intense effort. In truth, achievement and action needn't produce this stress. How do you manifest masculine energy? Are you able to achieve and still remain relaxed? Getting the job done while staying free and loose in your body requires that your action come from your core.[41]

Dr. Rolf's Words
Related to the Ninth Session

"You cannot experience true joint movement until it is initiated from the inside with intrinsic muscles. Any movement which is primarily extrinsic is only an approximation of true movement."[42]

"Work is the job of the sleeve, being is the job of the core."[43]

Practitioner Goals
for the Ninth Session

+ Release rotations in the upper half of the body.
+ Balance the superficial and deep muscles of the arms, shoulders, back, chest, neck, and head.
+ Organize the shoulder girdle and connect it to the lumbodorsal hinge.

Areas Addressed

The upper half of the body is the focus of this session. Areas addressed include the rib cage, arms, shoulders, and neck. By this point in the series, deeper strain may be surfacing in your shoulder girdle. It's time for your practitioner to help release any strain patterns or rotations in your upper body that may be preventing your shoulder girdle from resting squarely on top of your rib cage.

As you stand in front of a mirror, do you notice one shoulder being higher than the other or one hand and arm presenting more forward than the other? An asymmetry such as this can be caused by a twist in the rib cage that plays out in a three-dimensional rotation pattern of the upper back. Joseph Heller depicts this in the image of a water carrier with a pole across his shoulders and buckets at the end of it that are rotated forward and backward across his shoulders instead of resting squarely and evenly across it.[44]

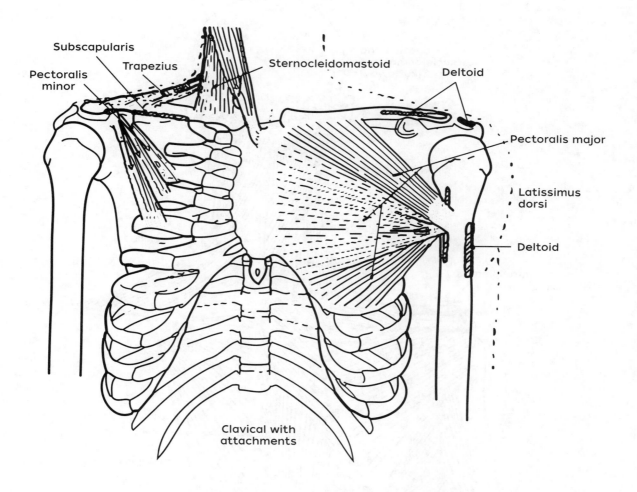

✦ Fig. 2.26. The superficial and deep musculature of the shoulder girdle (anterior).

From *Rolfing: Reestablishing the Natural Alignment and Structural Integration of the Human Body for Vitality and Well-Being* by Ida P. Rolf, Ph.D.
Reprinted with permission of publisher.

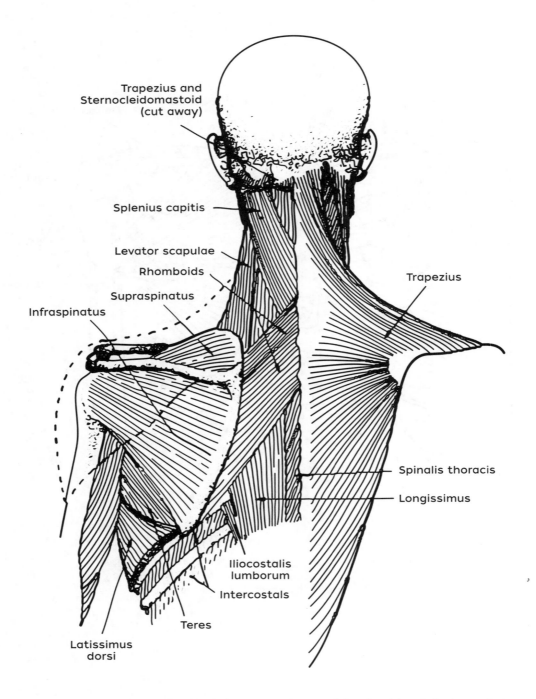

Trapezius and
Sternocleidomastoid
(cut away)

Splenius capitis

Levator scapulae

Rhomboids

Supraspinatus

Infraspinatus

Trapezius

Spinalis thoracis

Longissimus

Iliocostalis
lumborum

Intercostals

Teres

Latissimus
dorsi

✦ Fig. 2.27. The superficial and deep musculature of the shoulder girdle (posterior).

From *Rolfing: Reestablishing the Natural Alignment and Structural Integration
of the Human Body for Vitality and Well-Being* by Ida P. Rolf, Ph.D.
Reprinted with permission of publisher.

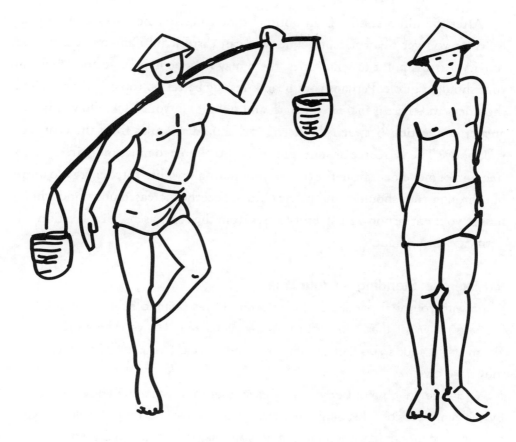

◆ Fig. 2.28. Rotated shoulder girdle shown carrying water (left)
and standing upright (right).

This drawing was adapted by Carolyn Cameron from the Hellerwork *Client's Handbook*
and used with kind permission of Hellerwork International, LLC.

The Energetics of
the Line in the Ninth Session

Dr. Rolf described the pelvic girdle and shoulder girdle as the working structures of the body. The core structure of the spine she considered to be the "beingness" of a person. She said that when the girdles are free of the core, energy flows from the core out through the girdles.

By now, the Line is becoming well established in your body. If you recognize and utilize the significance and power of the Line, it will affect how you move through your life both physically and energetically.

After the ninth session is an optimal time to review how to stand on your Line. As you get this basic principle, you can carry it into any movement and activity. At this point in your series, there may now be more ease and length in your shoulder girdle. Perhaps your head is resting better on top of your neck and shoulders and there is increased length and stability in your back. Do you notice greater connection between the pelvic and shoulder girdles from the center of your body? The vertebrae of your spine may also be able to move more freely. This freedom of movement from the core of your body allows life-force energy to move out through your shoulder and pelvic girdles. Feel the increased unity and wholeness in your entire body. As stability arises from the core, a sense of relaxation can permeate throughout.

ஃ Exercise: Standing on Your Line

Stand with your feet parallel and your second toes pointed straight ahead. Your feet are no wider than the width between your ears. Let your hips drop like a weight from your spine. Let the floor or Earth support you. Your knees are soft; they have give.

Organize your major body segments so that they stack one above the other. By the ninth session, this alignment should be easier and more familiar to you, as your practitioner has been organizing your major body segments so that their center of gravity is around your central Line.

Find the top of your head. Remember, it is the place where two lines drawn from the center of your ears to the top of your head would intersect. Your eyes and chin are horizontal to the plane of the Earth. Your shoulders rest with ease on top of the rib cage that supports them.

There is a sense of lift from your waist up, and yet the weight of your body from your hips down is dropping down through the front of your ankles toward the Earth. Above your ankles, your body is light because all of its weight is either being dropped into the Earth or lifting skyward through the top of your head. And yet there is an incredible sense of grounding through your feet. This is the experience of being on your Line. Can you sense that energetic quality of lift through the top of your head and at the same time feel how very grounded you are in your feet?

Your body can rest and be supported by what is beneath it. There is no need to pull up and away from what you are standing on. Let your body be supported. This allows your nervous system to rest. Let this sense of ease and well-being permeate your body and your whole being. Feel your capacity just to *BE*, and to be *NOW*. Completely connected, you can be congruent within your body, mind, emotions, and spirit.

Take a breath, and use it to run the energy from the Earth up through your feet, up the center of your legs, along the front side of your spine, and out the top of your head into the energy field around your body. Then let your body naturally exhale. In like manner, take another breath, and use it to pull in the energy from the stars through the top of your head. With your exhalation, send that energy down into every cell of your body and every aspect of your being. In this way, your body becomes a conduit of this life-force connection, charging and renewing like a living crystal.

Self-Care for the Client after the Ninth Session

Follow the suggestions for self-care that are outlined beginning on page 39, particularly taking a short walk immediately after your session and taking your first detox bath within six hours. Remember to drink plenty of water. As you walk, notice how freely your arms and legs can swing. Are both sides of your body moving similarly? Are there any areas that still feel stuck? See if you can feel your movement originating from the core of your body at the center of your spine.

Movement Awareness for the Client after the Ninth Session

This session is about creating more length and space in the shoulder girdle and then connecting that length into the core lumbar area with support from the lower body. A teacher of mine told me, "The hallmark of success for the eighth and ninth sessions is when you ask for movement and the client is able to perform the movement without shortening."

Now, as you go about your day, breathe fully into your rib cage and shoulder girdle. Own those spaces where breath can move more fully.

Heller notes that movement of the arms and legs works best when the core and the sleeve of the body are integrated. For example, when throwing a ball, if you throw it with just your arm, you'll be engaging primarily the outer sleeve muscles.

If you let the movement come from your core, your whole body will move. When you throw with your whole body, you'll also have more power in your arm movements and more stability in your stance.[45]

We want you to integrate the movement of the whole body—both core and sleeve. Notice the difference between the two types of movement. Throw a ball using just your arm. Then throw the ball from the core of your body, connecting that movement into your back and out through your arms. There is a big difference, isn't there? Take these principles of movement from your core and whole body movement into your daily activities, like office work, gardening, exercising, walking, playing a musical instrument, and so on.

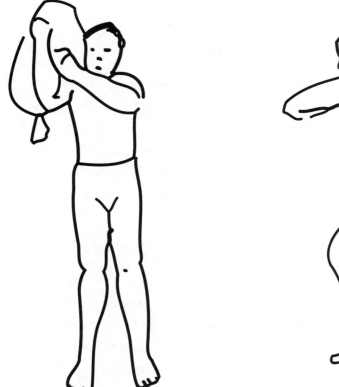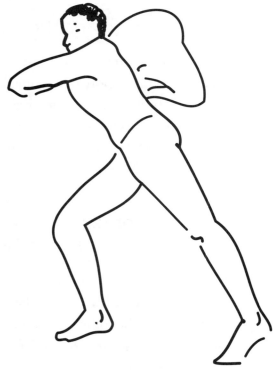

✦ Fig. 2.29. Shoulder girdle movement throwing from the outer sleeve (left)
and throwing from the core (right).

This drawing was adapted by Carolyn Cameron from the Hellerwork *Client's Handbook*
and used with kind permission of Hellerwork International, LLC.

Between the
Ninth and Tenth Sessions

From the Hellerwork perspective, the span between the ninth and tenth sessions is a time to focus on the connection between action and relaxation. Heller says, "Notice an area of your life that needs clear and penetrating action. Perform the necessary action with continued awareness and relaxation of your core. Notice how your body feels as you carry out this action. Remember to breathe and relax."[46]

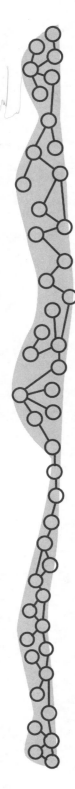

SESSION TEN
Integration

The Theme of the Tenth Session

Joseph Heller describes the theme of this session as "integration." He tells us:

> By this we mean revealing integrity that is already there—not adding anything new. We are simply uncovering the natural integrity and balance of the body. Integrity means wholeness, completeness and totality. It comes from the Latin word *integer,* which is derived from the verb *tegere,* which means "to touch." In that sense, integrity is the experience of being in touch with yourself and with your wholeness and completeness. Are you beginning to feel your own natural integrity? The joints, which are the main bodily focus of this session, reflect maturity—children have unstable joints, and older people have rigid joints. A stable but freely moving joint is an expression of maturity. In that sense, this session is the embodiment of growing up.[47]

Dr. Rolf's Words
Related to the Tenth Session

"Thanks to the fasciae and the physical properties of its collagen, we have been able to shift one unit atop another—pelvis above leg, thorax over pelvis, and neck and head on the top. In so doing, we have greatly improved the mechanical stacking of these structural units, but this is not basically a mechanical system. It is a living system within a gravitational field; therefore, it is an electrical system, a polar system."[48]

"True verticality, the goal of Structural Integration, is more than a figment of the imagination. Indeed, it is very real; it is a functional phenomenon, a line around which the body's energy force fields balance. . . . Through its vertical stance, the organism is no longer earth-bound; the vertical expresses an energy relation between earth and sun."[49]

Practitioner Goals for
the Tenth Session

✦ Balance and stabilize the joints of the body.

✦ Establish even, balanced tone and span within the layers of the myofascial tissues. "Good tone" equates to healthy chemical balance in the tissues. The body also lengthens as it gets better tone. "Good span" describes adequate and balanced spatial arrangement of the tissues. With good tone and span, the structure of the body has balance. The connective tissues can respond quickly and easily to any situation, be they at rest or at work.

Areas Addressed

The areas addressed in this session include all the major joints of the body; that is, the ankles, knees, hips, shoulders, elbows, wrists, neck, and spine. The joint spaces are an integral part of connecting the major body segments and balancing them within the gravitational field. Now we want to stabilize these joints and free them of any remaining rotation. When we create length and space within the myofascial tissues around the joints, the body segments can move as freely as possible.

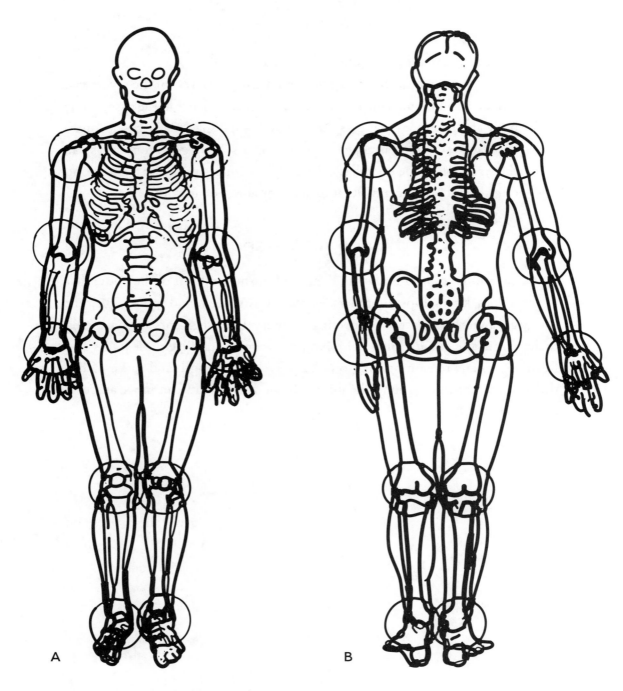

✦ Fig. 2.30. Skeletal system with joints circled: (A) anterior; (B) posterior.

This drawing was adapted by Carolyn Cameron from the Hellerwork *Client's Handbook* and used with kind permission of Hellerwork International, LLC.

The Energetics of the Line in the Tenth Session

The following words are from "Free Balance," a poem by Richard Podolny, a Rolfing practitioner who is also board certified in family medicine and holistic medicine:

> *Structural Integration is the balancing of a human body in three dimensional space. It is the evoking of the innate connection within all human beings, with the Earth and the Heavens, with the Mother and the Father, with the Source and the Sourceless. . . .*
>
> *A body that has been Structurally Integrated manifests a line, an open core that allows life to move through it, and manifest from it, in infinite directions. . . .*
>
> *Structural Integration is freeing muscles to move independently. Freeing bones to allow themselves to go naturally into place. Freeing nerves to flow the information of life without interference. Freeing the spirit to move as it will and having the courage to move with it.*
>
> *How much fear could you possibly feel if, just by standing, you could sense the whole earth supporting and lifting you towards the heavens. This is being balanced. It is being Structurally Integrated.*

Such a powerful description of this transformational process! The physical body *is* the composite of the mental, emotional, and spiritual selves. Significant work in any of those aspects of a person's being will have its effect on the others. This is the experience of Structural Integration. People surprise themselves and others with how much they change during this process.

People of all ages and walks of life benefit from Structural Integration, particularly those who have had car accidents resulting in whiplash. People look taller, thinner, and almost always younger. Older folks often get the spring back in their step and walk with more grace. "George, you came straight!" a friend exclaimed after one of my older clients completed his Structural Integration series. Another client, Barbara, looked like she had lost considerable weight, but the scale remained the same. She was incredulous when we discovered that she had gained more than an inch in height! Mary Sue, a woman in her late sixties, lost her dowager's hump and got her head back on top of her shoulders. She also gained full cervical range

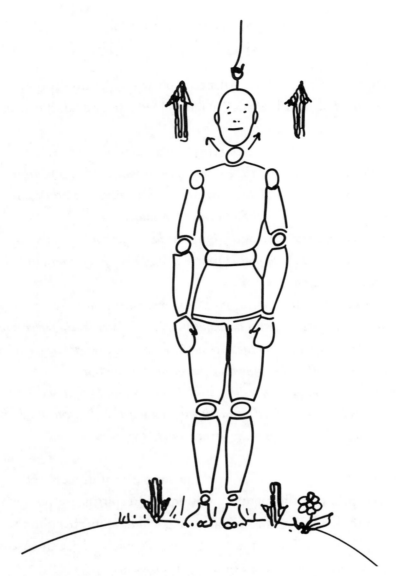

✦ Fig. 2.31. The body on the Line suspended between the Earth and sky.
This drawing was adapted by Carolyn Cameron from the Hellerwork *Client's Handbook* and used with kind permission of Hellerwork International, LLC.

of motion with her series. People who hadn't seen her for a while said that she looked fifteen years younger!

It is my joy in sharing this work to see people springboard from Structural Integration into a new phase in their lives. As they let go of the old that does not serve, they step into and own who they are NOW. This work has helped give many people the self-confidence, motivation, and self-awareness they need to make the next step in their lives and careers. That's what can happen naturally when strain in the body is cleared!

Self-Care for the Client after the Tenth Session

Follow the suggestions for self-care that are outlined beginning on page 39, particularly taking a short walk immediately after your session and taking your first detox bath within six hours. Remember to drink plenty of water.

Now, having completed the ten-session series, take some time for reflection. Spend some time under the stars. Lie on the Earth. Contemplate your Structural Integration Journey. You may want to pull out the list you made at the beginning of your series and appreciate how far you have come. Know that the changes you have experienced and the lessons you have learned are yours, and they will continue to work for you in the times ahead.

Movement Awareness for the Client after the Tenth Session

Structural Integration is a dynamic process for dynamic human beings. Within this work, we have intended to bring order out of disorganized body segments and create a new level of structural and functional wholeness; one that you can take with you and work with in your own life. Balance of body, mind, emotion, and spirit is an ongoing process and worthy of being gentle with one's self. In this final tenth session, your practitioner has addressed the joints of your body for their optimal balance so that movement can be initiated from the core of your body.

⚛ Exercise: Core Breathing

Lie on your back with your knees up against your chest. Wrap your arms around your knees to totally relax your lower back. Let go of your stomach muscles. Let go of any holding at your pelvic floor or shoulders. Keep your chin down, and reach long through the top of your head to lengthen your spine. Breathe as deeply as you can into your ribs. Breathe into your pelvic floor. Feel the floor of your pelvis moving with every breath. Release any holding there. By doing this, you can help your entire nervous system relax. Move your breath along the entire length of your spine. You are connected from the top down and the bottom up. Any strain in one end can affect the other. So too, the release of strain in one end can help bring ease and relaxation to the other.

⚇ Exercise: Moving from a Place of Connection

With attention along your energetic Line, imagine a skyhook at the top of your head, gently lifting you upward. Feel the lengthening of the segments between your spine and neck with this subtle suspension. Feel the gentle pull of gravity from the Earth. This subtle suspension allows your shoulders to rest on your rib cage and your arms to release at your sides. With alignment of your body segments, all of your body weight can drop into the Earth. Stacked body segments in alignment = stable structure. Sense this more stable connection with the Earth along with the feeling of lift from above. In this way, the body becomes a living conduit between the forces of the heavens and the Earth.

With this feeling of lift from the skyhook and grounding to the Earth, connect into your Line that runs along the front of your spine and extends into the heavens and Earth. Move from that place of connection. Walk with awareness of your Line. Can you feel the lift and ease between your joints? How does that feel? It is possible to experience your entire body moving as an integrated whole. Enjoy the flow and ease of such connected movement.[50]

After the Tenth Session

After the conclusion of my own first experience of Structural Integration, I remember feeling a strong sense of my own ability to achieve my dreams and goals. That series led me to become a practitioner, and what a path of awareness this has been! In my early days of training, Emmett said that the path of a practitioner of this work was a path of awareness. I asked him what he meant. "You'll see," he said with his usual smile.

A client of mine asked me what she should do after her tenth session. I replied, "Learn to live on your Line."

In the last moments of Dr. Rolf's life, Emmett asked her, "Who is going to be my teacher when you are gone?" Dr. Rolf looked at him and said,

"Your Line will be your teacher!"

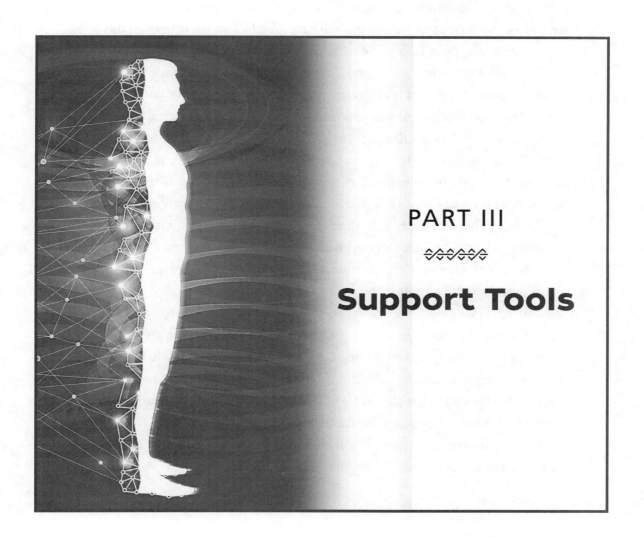

PART III

❖❖❖❖❖

Support Tools

We human beings are both physical and energetic beings. The body is the container that holds our mental, emotional, and spiritual selves. Significant change in any one of those aspects of our being will have an effect on the others. In this way, our energetic blueprint informs our physical body.

Dr. Rolf knew that Structural Integration is a transformational process. Organizing body structure and clearing stress and strain from the connective tissue is paramount for the flow of beneficial life-force energy. When that energy is able to flow, a more evolved and aware human being may emerge.

So as we proceed into this wonderful possibility through the process of Structural Integration, we could ask the following questions: What is stress? Where does it come from? How can we minimize stress and strain in the body?

Stress can be defined as a detrimental force that interferes with the normal physiological equilibrium of an organism. When the force of stress is internalized in the body, it is known as strain. Strain is internalized stress.

Where does stress come from? It has a plethora of physical, mental, and emotional origins. Consider the accidents, injuries, and emotional traumas that are part of the human experience. Such experiences leave an imprint in the body. Those physical, mental, and emotional imprints of stress are what Structural Integrators strive to remove. With such clearing and balancing, people become more internally and externally aware of perceptions within and around them. In doing so, understanding arises. Better choices become available.

In the following chapters, we will look at the support tools that can help us minimize the forces of stress in the body and optimize our human experience.

THE BEMER

My Journey with the Heavenly and Earthly Energies

On a November day in 2008, while I was doing paperwork at the Chico Sports Club, an occupational therapist named Jan Condon recommended that I try her BEMER. She described it as a therapeutic mat that resonated a pulsed electromagnetic field. I was intrigued by her description, so I tried it.

To my surprise, her electromagnetic device produced waves of energy in my body that were very similar to the ones I was already familiar with from my meditation practices. I called those sensations "heavenly and earthly energies." For years I had felt these waves without the aid of any technology, and here I was having a very similar experience with an electromagnetic device. Amazing!

I first noticed the heavenly energy that flows into my body through the top of my head when I was sixteen, after reading *Autobiography of a Yogi* by Paramahansa Yogananda. That book began my spiritual quest and practice of meditation.

In February 1984, those waves of heavenly energy became much stronger in me. I was in northern India in the village of Haidakhan Vishwa Mahadham, at the ashram of Haidakhan Babaji. This place is described in Sanskrit as "the holiest place in the universe." I had come to meet Babaji, whom Yogananda referred to as "the Immortal Yogi." Babaji is said to appear through the ages for the benefit of mankind. I had traveled far on my own, pulled by the desire to meet him.

While sitting in view of the Ganges River, next to a *duni* (a ceremonial fire pit made of clay and cow dung in which a continuous fire burned), I suddenly felt strong waves of tingling energy pour in through the top of my head and rush up and down my spine. It felt wonderful!

In my mind's eye, those waves of energy looked like showers of brilliant specks of light that lit me up from inside. I sensed that the fundamental essence of those energies was Love and that every cell of my body was fed by those waves of energy.

I had known this sensation before, but never as strongly as I did on that day in Haidakhan. From then on, those sensations became much more familiar to me.

Now my body has learned to resonate with them. Sometimes I draw the energies into me just by focusing my attention on them. At other times they occur spontaneously.

Several years later, in 1987, while practicing a form of body-centered awareness called Vipassana meditation, I had my first experience of earthly energy that moved into my body through the bottoms of my feet. I was sitting in a straight-backed chair in a home along the Hamakua coast of the Big Island of Hawaii. My feet were flat on the floor. I was paying attention to the movement of my breath when a tingling sensation began to stir in my feet. With each inhalation, I noticed the tingling moved farther up my legs, into my hips and then into my spine. It seemed like my breath was a pump that was moving the energy upward. Those sensations felt very similar to the heavenly energy, but they were moving into my body upward from the bottoms of my feet, so I called them earthly energy.

Through the years, I've noticed that these energies have different qualities. Through studies in energy medicine, I have learned that heavenly energy is more masculine and has a positive electrical charge. The earthly energy is more feminine and has a negative charge. Both are needed for balance. I have been guided to use them in different ways to help energize myself and to clear blockages in my physical, mental, and emotional bodies.

People are amazed at my stamina and energy level with the type and amount of work I do as a Rolf practitioner. I tell them I am accessing larger fields of energy that I consciously run through my body. That's what being on my Rolf Line is about. My body is not the exception. It is possible for all. It is our birthright to be connected in such a way.

I have often wondered how the natural energy flows I experience affect my physiology. Could they be similar to the benefits of the BEMER, which have been well researched and documented? I think so. Could the BEMER help other people learn to run energy through their body, even to the point of being able to do so without the aid of a technological device? Perhaps so. Maybe it can strengthen a person's living-matrix pathways where the meridians are embedded in the fascia, supporting the flow of life-force energy through the body.

For me, the BEMER does not replace the benefits derived from a regular meditation practice, but it does enhance the flow of life force through my body and my overall well-being.

What Is the BEMER?

BEMER stands for bio-electro-magnetic energy regulation, with the key word being *regulation*. This device pulses and regulates the intensity of electromagnetic energy through the body. It was developed in 1992 at a German university by Wolf Kafka, a German physicist and physiologist.

The BEMER's benefits to human physiology are well documented by scientific research. Clinical studies at the Institute of Microcirculation in Berlin have shown that the BEMER enhances *all* metabolic processes in the body. Other studies have shown that the BEMER increases circulation and energy production in the body. It can enhance the immune system, support the autonomic nervous system, and aid organ and skeletal structure through the support of the production of specific proteins that our bodies need.

The Significance of Electromagnetic Fields to the Human Body

The importance of electromagnetic fields to our bodies became clear in the 1970s when we first sent astronauts into space. After twenty-four hours in space, the astronauts returned to Earth with "space sickness"; that is, energy depletion and a lack of strength. NASA researchers concluded that the astronauts had suffered because they were out of range of the electromagnetic field of the earth. The scientists realized that the Earth's electromagnetic field is vital to us. Not only does the field protect us from radiation, it is also necessary for proper physiological function of the body. As a result of studies from early space travel, space suits and capsules are now equipped with magnetic field generators of 50 microtesla that simulate electromagnetic fields of the Earth.[1]

During her time in the physics department at UCLA in the 1970s, Valerie Hunt demonstrated the importance of electromagnetic fields to our bodies through her creation of the Mu Room—a small room where the natural electromagnetic energy of the air could be altered without changing the level of gravitational force or the oxygen content. Researchers "could also direct electromagnetic frequencies to and from various locations in the room." When the Mu Room was flooded with electromagnetic energy, subjects experienced enhanced coordination, high levels of consciousness, and a sense of well-being. When the electromagnetism in the room was depleted, subjects fell apart emotionally and experienced a loss of their physical coordination and their intellectual abilities.[2]

Through such studies, some scientists have determined that the electromagnetic field of the Earth is critical for the proper functioning and survival of our bodies. All life on this planet has evolved under the influence of this field.

Energy Production and Cellular Metabolism

"Every single ailment starts with a lack of circulation and oxygen," said Horst Michaelis, MD, in his talk at Dominican University. Insufficient circulation and oxygen diminishes the body's ability to produce ATP. The ATP molecule supplies the energy that our cells need to maintain themselves. If ATP production is down, cells can't live out their life cycle and will die prematurely, creating chronically degenerative conditions. Insufficient circulation also contributes to poor immune health, which contributes to the development of degenerative conditions and diseases.

ATP is produced by mitochondria, which are found, along with other organelles, in the cytoplasm of the body's cells. The body has to make energy continuously; at any one time, there is only one to two seconds' worth of reserve energy in the body. Dr. Michaelis explained that the pulsed electromagnetic field of the BEMER has been shown to boost ATP production by the mitochondria, giving the body more energy at a cellular level.

The energy created by ATP production also helps maintain the proper voltage across cell membranes; without proper voltage in red blood cells, the membranes collapse. Red blood cells repulse each other when they have sufficient electrical charge. When they are deficient in voltage, they start attracting each other and clump together. When clumped, blood cells become too thick to pass through the tiny capillaries where nutrients and oxygen are delivered into the cells and waste is taken away. High blood pressure can result. However, within eight to ten minutes after a person has been on the BEMER, clumped blood cells separate and flow more easily. More oxygen will be carried into the tissues as circulation of the blood at the capillary level is increased. Research with dark field microscopy shows an increase in circulation at the capillary level and an increase in oxygen with the use of the BEMER.*

The BEMER also causes white blood cells to slow down—to amble their way along the vessel walls, rather than racing by—and enables them to deal with pathogens and toxic substances more effectively.

The BEMER Signal

Life force is synonymous with electromagnetic frequencies. The BEMER pulses an electromagnetic field that resonates with our innate life-force energy. Electromagnetic fields have a wave pattern. The *frequency* of the wave describes the number of times it repeats per second. The pulsating electromagnetic waves of the BEMER are a broad-spectrum signal that includes sine waves of varying frequency. The broad-spectrum nature of the signal is important because the different cells of the body respond to different frequencies due to their different densities.

As we learned in part 1, the force of a magnetic field is measured in units known as tesla. The BEMER's pulsed magnetic field measures between 10 and 30 microtesla, which resonates well with the electromagnetic field of the Earth.

BEMER Components

BEMER technology has continued to advance through the years. My older BEMER 3000 model includes a mat with copper coils running through it. The mat plugs into a control unit. On the electrical cord between the wall outlet and the control unit is a transformer that converts AC current to DC current. The DC current flows through the copper coils in the mat, creating an electromagnetic field. The electromagnetic field emitted from the BEMER 3000 mat

---

*Research studies documenting the improvement of increased oxygen levels and fluidity of the blood using the BEMER can be found in the Academy for Bioenergetics (AFB) publication "Technical Information: BEMER-3000 Therapy," at http://www.innomed.co.za/bemer3000/dls/AFB-eng .pdf.

extends 16 inches above and below the mat. As the current is increased or decreased through settings on the control unit, the magnetic field will increase or decrease accordingly.

It is significant that the BEMER uses pulsating direct current. In alternating current (AC), the electrons reverse their direction at regularly occurring intervals. In direct current (DC), the electrons flow only in one direction. The electromagnetic field of the Earth operates on DC current. The cells of our bodies only recognize and benefit from direct current. This type of current supports human physiology.

The control unit allows the user to vary the intensity of the electromagnetic signal. The signal generally runs for eight to ten minutes. The unit may also have programs that run for up to twenty minutes and are designed to help increase vasomotion, which is the contraction and expansion of the arterial walls. Our bodies use this contraction and expansion of the blood vessel walls to move blood to areas of the body where it is needed.

The signal can also travel into a smaller device called an intensive applicator. The intensive applicator is used for deeper penetrative effects on local areas.

Using the BEMER

The BEMER is designed to be used three or four times a day with an interval of three to four hours between uses. If it is used only twice a day, users are advised to double the length of application. The BEMER will support rest and repair of the body or the increase of energy production if needed.

I love to use the BEMER as a restorative "nap machine." If I want to drop into a parasympathetic state of rest and repair, I put the BEMER on its lowest setting and quickly drop into a productive twelve-minute session. I feel relaxed and ready to go again when the session is complete.

If my energy level is lower than I would like, I set the BEMER on its highest setting and relax on the mat. During that time, I will feel the pulsed electromagnetic energy move through my body, knowing it is upgrading the various systems in my body as needed.

I'll have my clients lie on the BEMER after a particularly challenging session. Putting the BEMER on its lowest setting supports their parasympathetic nervous system. After a few minutes of rest, their body will integrate and they will be ready to head out the door.

The BEMER has been a great tool in my life and in my Structural Integration practice. I am grateful to have it. For more information on the BEMER, see united-states.bemergroup.com.

FAR-INFRARED SAUNA

The far-infrared sauna is another electromagnetic healing device that has been particularly helpful for some of my Structural Integration clients. I recommend it for clients who have persisting soreness for more than several days after a session, even after having done their detox baths. A far-infrared sauna will provide a more thorough detox for their body. By using the sauna, a person can quickly sweat and efficiently eliminate toxins that have been stirred up in their tissues from the bodywork. These toxins are generally the source of soreness.

What Is Far-Infrared?

Far-infrared radiation is the warm, gentle radiant heat that comes from the sun. Approximately 80 percent of the sun's energy is far-infrared rays. Infrared is a band of light on the electromagnetic spectrum, not visible to the naked eye. The specific wavelength of light for infrared rays measures between 750 nanometers and 100 micrometers.[3]

Far-infrared waves heat objects without having to heat the air around them. This process is called conversion. The waves cause molecules in an object to vibrate against each other, producing heat. Because of this, the far-infrared saunas operate at a much lower temperature than a conventional sauna.

The waves of far-infrared can penetrate up to 1.5 inches beneath the skin. This deep penetration causes vibrations of proteins, collagen, fat, and water molecules in muscular tissues and internal organs. The heat produced by these vibrations raises body temperature, causing dilation of blood vessels, increased heart rate, increased blood circulation, and a strong sweating response in the body.[4]

Here are a few of the many benefits of far-infrared saunas:

+ Detoxification of gases, heavy metals, and other toxins held in the body's fat[5]
+ Reduction of blood pressure as a result of dilation of the blood vessels[6]
+ Inhibiting of the proliferation of some cancer cells such as breast, lung, and tongue through change in body temperature[7]

✦ Aiding in the treatment of chronic ailments and medical conditions such as diabetes, cardiovascular disease, congestive heart failure, chronic fatigue, rheumatoid arthritis, depression, anger management issues, poor digestion, and chronic muscle and joint pain[8]

To optimize results with a far-infrared sauna:

✦ Set the sauna temperature to between 100°F and 140°F.
✦ Exercise for ten to thirty minutes before using the sauna to help release toxins.
✦ Drink plenty of water before and after the sauna.
✦ Shower before the sauna to increase sweating.
✦ Remain in the sauna for a minimum of fifteen to twenty minutes.
✦ Sit in different places during the sauna to heat your body evenly.
✦ Drink an electrolyte-rich drink, such as the Himalayan salt sole (page 131), after the sauna to replace minerals released through sweating.
✦ Rinse off in a warm or cool shower after the sauna to remove toxins.

Contraindications: If you feel dizzy, become nauseous, or get a headache during the sauna, leave the sauna. The next time you use the sauna, try less time and less heat. You may have to work up to a full-strength sauna.

People with multiple sclerosis, lupus, hemophilia, or injuries less than forty-eight hours old should avoid the far-infrared sauna. Women who are breastfeeding or pregnant should also avoid it. When in doubt, consult with a physician.

THE ROLE OF NUTRITION

Having done bodywork for years, I've seen people come into my office with a variety of ailments besides their structural problems and injuries. These conditions may include fibromyalgia, chronic fatigue, high cholesterol, excessive weight, osteoarthritis or rheumatoid arthritis, allergies, inflammation, pain and stiffness in joints and tissues, acid reflux, osteoporosis, and bone spurs. I've noticed a common denominator across many of these conditions: congestion, stiffness, and inflammation in the tissues and joints. These conditions, I believe, based on my own studies and healing journey, are linked to nutrition and, more specifically, to an overload of acidic toxins that have backed up in the connective tissues.

While nutrition is not my expertise, it has been a significant part of my personal journey. I share the following information with my clients, and I offer it to you for your well-being and consideration.

The Importance of Salt

Many people are under the impression that salt is not good for us. In truth, salt is a vital nutrient for our body. While some people do indeed need to limit salt in their diet due to their particular constitution, for most of us, the determining factor in whether or not salt is good for us is what *kind* of salt it is.

All salts are not equal. Some have been highly processed with extreme heat and many chemical processes that strip them of minerals. Such salt *is* bad for us. It is very difficult for the body to eliminate.

Unprocessed or "raw" salt remains whole, mineral rich, and alkaline. It contains sodium, chloride, potassium, calcium, and magnesium, as well as many trace minerals. Many of these constituents function as electrolytes; that is, they conduct electrical energy to the cells and help maintain hydration, blood pH, and nerve and muscle function. (Processed salts, in contrast, cannot conduct electrical energy.)[9] The abundant magnesium in unprocessed salt helps balance the sodium content so it won't raise blood pressure. Such healthy alkalizing salt is an essential part of our daily diet and necessary for proper function of the body.

In my bodywork, I encourage clients to make Himalayan salt sole, a concentrated electrolyte-rich solution of pink Himalayan salt, and drink a small amount of it daily, diluted in pure water. When they use this sole regularly, I've noticed that arthritic tissues and joints clear more quickly and thoroughly, making my work with them much easier.

⚘ Making Himalayan Salt Sole

Fill a quart glass jar with 1 pound of Himalayan pink salt. Add 1 quart of filtered water. Let the mixture sit for twenty-four hours; then it's ready. Every day, shake the bottle well, then pour off anywhere from ¼ teaspoon to 1 teaspoon of the salty brine into an 8-ounce glass of filtered water, and drink. The sole mixture does not need to be refrigerated.

The sole will help alkalize the pH of the body and remove toxins from the tissues and joints. Start slowly, using the lower end of the dosage range and increasing gradually, up to one teaspoon. Back off if symptoms of detox become uncomfortable.

Pink Himalayan salt, hand-harvested unprocessed Celtic sea salt, and Real Salt, a commercial brand harvested from deposits in Utah, are examples of good-quality raw salts. Biophysicist James Oschman also highly recommends Quinton Marine Plasma, a seawater tonic that contains amino acids, fatty acids, and a full spectrum of mineral salts.

The Body and pH

In the term *pH,* the *p* stands for "power" and *H* is the symbol for the element hydrogen. The pH of a solution describes its degree of acidity or alkalinity according to a logarithmic scale from 1 to 14, where 7 is the neutral pH of pure water. Numbers less than 7 express acidity, and numbers greater than 7 express alkalinity. Each whole pH number below 7 is ten times more acidic than the number above it. And each whole pH number above 7 is ten times more alkaline than the number below it.

Just as the body, in homeostasis, works to maintain a constant temperature of 98.6°F, it also works to keep the pH of the blood in an alkaline range between 7.35 and 7.45 pH. If it strays outside this range, the pH is acidic and may damage tissues and organs.

You can measure your own body's pH using test strips available at any pharmacy. Test your first morning urine after 4:00 a.m., following the instructions that come with the test strip. The pH should register between 6.8 and 7.2 for optimal balance.

Dietary Factors

One of the primary factors that affect the pH of the body is our diet. Every food or drink we consume is metabolized and "burned," leaving a residual ash that is either acidic or alkaline. The pH of the food before it is consumed is not an indication of its effect on the body's pH. Citrus fruits, for example, like lemons, limes, and grapefruits, have an acidic pH of around 2.8, but once they are "burned" in the body they leave an alkaline ash.[10] On the other hand, all vinegars remain acidic before and after being metabolized.

In their book *The pH Miracle: Balance Your Diet, Reclaim Your Health,* nutritionist and microbiologist Robert Young and massage therapist and chef Shelley Redford Young state, "The human body is alkaline by design and acidic by function. What that means in practice is that the body needs alkaline fuel and that acid wastes are naturally created as a by-product of all human activity."[11]

The trouble begins when too many acid toxins overload our systems. "A chronically overacidic pH corrodes body tissue, and interrupts all cellular activity from the beating of the heart to the neural firing of the brain and leads to sickness and disease," state Young and Young.[12]

The Body's Defenses against Acidic Toxins

The liver and kidneys form the first line of defense against excessive acidity in the body. However, a diet high in acid foods such as meat, dairy, grains, high-sugar fruit, and bread may exceed the capacity of the liver and kidneys to filter acidic toxins. Those toxins will then back up into the connective tissues, creating inflammation and potential damage to organs and tissues. The following information describes the mechanisms through which the body protects against, neutralizes, or removes acidic toxins through fat, cholesterol, and minerals.

+ **Fat.** Some of the acids will be stored in fat to keep them from negatively affecting vital internal organs. Young and Young tell us, "It has been shown that the body holds onto fat to protect itself from an overacidic condition."[13]

An overly acidic pH over a prolonged period of time will impede the body's ability to absorb essential vitamins and minerals. They go on to say, "Neither nutrients from food nor supplements can be absorbed in an acid environment. . . . This weakens the body's ability to produce enzymes and hormones. It also interferes with reconstruction of cells and energy production, creating fatigue and general weakness."[14]

✦ **Cholesterol.** The liver releases cholesterol to neutralize acidic toxins. However, when a person takes drugs to reduce cholesterol without reducing the input of excessive acids into his or her system, it could be "a recipe for disaster," state Young and Young. As acid levels rise in the body, so does the cholesterol level and the risk for stroke and heart attack.[15]

✦ **Minerals.** "Minerals in general rule over other nutrients because vitamins, enzymes, and amino acids, as well as fats and carbohydrates require them for activity," states Mark Sircus, Ac., OMD.[16] The body uses base minerals, including sodium, potassium, calcium, and magnesium, to neutralize strong acids. If our diets do not contain enough minerals, the body will pull minerals from itself—sodium and potassium from blood plasma, calcium from bones and teeth, magnesium from muscles, and so on—to neutralize the acids and assist their elimination from the body. But this may rob the body of its own mineral stores, leading directly to bone loss, arthritis, and tooth decay.[17]

Once these minerals have been used to neutralize acidic pH, they have to be reabsorbed back into the bones at the junction of the tendon and bone. With prolonged acidic pH, the constant movement of minerals back and forth from the bones to the blood, along with their poor reabsorption, causes minerals to get stuck at the joints, creating arthritis, inflammation, pain, and reduced energetic and physiological flow.

An Ode to Magnesium

Magnesium has truly been a miracle mineral in my life! I used to suffer from chronic constipation. I also had such severe cramping in my hands and forearms that I wondered if I would be able to continue doing bodywork. After one 400 mg dose of Solaray Magnesium Asporotate, I was absolutely delighted to experience an easy morning bowel movement and the gradual release of contraction in my hands and arms!

Calcium causes contraction, and magnesium releases it. The more physically active we are, the greater our need for magnesium. The body doesn't produce it, so we have to take it in through our food and supplements. Foods high in magnesium include pumpkin seeds, almonds, sesame seeds, walnuts, and dark leafy greens.

Magnesium is needed for at least three hundred different biochemical processes in the body, including the metabolism of carbohydrates, fats, and amino acids. It helps the body with the following functions:

- ✦ Maintains nerve and muscle function
- ✦ Regulates blood sugar
- ✦ Stabilizes heart rate
- ✦ Relaxes the nervous system and helps keep cortisol levels low
- ✦ Helps create energy in the body
- ✦ Supports immune function
- ✦ Supports cognitive function
- ✦ Promotes the formation of bones and teeth
- ✦ Prevents calcification of organs and tissues
- ✦ Fosters deep and prolonged sleep

According to Merrily Kuhn, RN, Ph.D., practicing naturopathic physician and leading seminar presenter in continuing education programs in the United States, 60 to 80 percent of Americans are magnesium deficient. Kuhn suggests a dosage of up to 1,000 mg of magnesium daily.[18]

A Dietary Goal

The goal for the body is to be in an anabolic or alkaline state of regeneration, rather than a catabolic or acidic state of degeneration. The way to do that is by eating a balance of alkaline and acid foods.

According to Young and Young, ideally 80 percent of our diet would be alkaline foods and 20 percent would be healthy acidic foods. The healthy acidic foods would include whole grains, beans, wild-caught fish, and pasture-raised, hormone- and antibiotic-free lean meats. The alkaline foods would include vegetables, soaked and sprouted nuts and seeds, unprocessed salts, low-sugar fruits and alkaline water.[19]

Alkaline Water

The health of our connective tissue is affected by the level of our hydration. Alkaline water with a pH between 9 and 11 not only hydrates the connective tissues but also gently neutralizes and removes acid wastes from the body. Young and Young described the importance of alkaline water: "For optimal health, your water must be energized-saturated with electrons. Water like that is highly charged and full of potential energy. It's also alkaline. In fact, water is alkaline because of the negative charge from all its electrons. Acids are dominated by positively charged protons. It is the attraction of electrons to protons that allows alkaline substances to neutralize acidic substances."[20]

"Water molecules cluster together when they lose their electrical charge. All acidic water has larger molecular clusters."[21] That includes tap water and bottled water. Water with larger molecular clusters has difficulty being absorbed through cell membranes. I myself noticed a period of time when no matter how much water I drank, I wasn't feeling hydrated. That's because the acidic water I was drinking lacked minerals and had larger molecular clusters that my body could not absorb. I changed my water filter to one that alkalized the water, added beneficial minerals, created smaller water molecule clusters, and put an electrical charge into the water. Then I had the satisfaction and benefit of feeling hydrated. (The Nikken Aqua Pour gravity water system and AlkaViva Elita countertop water ionizer have worked well for me.)

Chlorophyll

Chlorophyll has been called the "blood of plants." Its molecular structure is the same as human blood except its central atom is magnesium. Young and Young call green juices, which are full of chlorophyll, "the superstars of the nutrition world" and note that chlorophyll helps build blood by improving the quality and quantity of red blood cells.[22]

Raw Foods vs. Cooked Foods

Foods usually become more acidic when cooked. Acid foods require neutralization through the electrons stored in the minerals of the body. Young and Young recommend that of the alkaline foods we eat, half of them should be eaten raw, because raw alkaline foods are abundant in electrons. "Electrons are, in fact, what make them alkaline. This is the energy the body runs on," they state.[23] If you must cook your food, do so for as short a time as possible. "Heat over 118° Fahrenheit destroys the electrical potential in food."[24] Organic food is best, of course, and all produce should be eaten as fresh as possible.

Young and Young suggest having your largest meal of the day at breakfast and then tapering off food intake by dinner to minimize an overload of acids before sleep and to allow the body to focus its energies on regeneration, rather than digestion, at night.[25]

"As a person eats more alkalizing foods, especially raw vegetables and greens," they say, "there is an extreme improvement in red blood cell integrity, oxygenation of the blood, levels of acidity, and negative microforms."[26]

Combating Microforms

Harmful microscopic organisms called microforms thrive in an overly acidic body when a low oxygen level occurs in the blood. Microforms include bacteria, yeasts, molds, and fungi, including candida, that produce very acidic toxins themselves. These microforms live off the food we eat that would have given our body energy. They also rob the body of important vitamins and minerals, compromising its ability to function.[27]

Foods that are high in sugar feed such beasties. For this reason, it is a good idea to avoid excessive sweet fruits and carbohydrates like white rice, white bread, white potatoes, and bananas. "Healthy tissue requires slow burning, low sugar 'green' foods for optimal wellness," states Deborah Page Johnson, author of *Home Test pH Kit*.[28]

Low-oxygen environments also support microforms. "If you can keep your blood clean and well oxygenated," states Johnson, "viruses, parasites and abnormal cells will have an inhospitable environment. Without oxygen they proliferate, with oxygen they die."[29] The health of the body is in the health of the blood.

The Importance of Gut Bacteria

I attended a seminar sponsored by the Institute for Brain Potential in Chico, California, where Dr. Kuhn presented. The title of her seminar was Understanding the Gut Brain: Stress, Appetite, Digestion, and Mood. She spoke extensively about the significance of gut bacteria. Here's what I learned.

Three to 4 pounds of bacteria live in the guts. They synthesize vitamins, produce hormones and digestive enzymes to absorb minerals, and play a part in the body's immune function. (The gut contains 70 to 90 percent of the body's immune cells.) These microorganisms, together with those found everywhere else, from our skin to our eyelashes, comprise as much as 90 percent of the cells in and on our bodies—a staggering percentage!

The bacteria in the gut can be categorized as "good" (that is, beneficial to humans) and "bad" (that is, harmful to humans). A proper ratio of gut bacteria would be 90 percent good bacteria and 10 percent bad bacteria. Good bacteria stimulate the immune and digestive systems, generate vitamins, help the body absorb nutrients, and provide a barrier to pathogens, which keeps the lining of the GI tract intact in order to prevent leaks. Sometimes we can experience an overgrowth of bad bacteria. This condition, known as dysbiosis, can lead to diarrhea and a host of other problems.

Leaky Gut

Among their other functions, the good bacteria in the gut provide a barrier against irritants that might otherwise damage the lining of the gastrointestinal (GI) tract. These include everything from pathogens and environmental toxins to additives, preservatives, and genetically modified foods. When our population of good bacteria is less than optimal, these irritants are able to damage the GI tract, causing inflammation.

Inflamed intestinal tissue allows leakage into the bloodstream of large undigested proteins, toxins, and bacteria. This can lead to further intestinal inflammation, malnutrition, food sensitivities, and bacterial and yeast overgrowths. Unsprouted grains, genetically modified organisms (GMOs), and hybridized foods contain large amounts of phytates and lectins. Phytates are the phosphorous compounds around a plant that act as a preservative until the plant is ready to germinate. In the human body, phytates act as antinutrients that bind to minerals, making the minerals unavailable to the body. Lectins are carbohydrate-binding proteins that cause cells and molecules to stick together. Lectins can attach to the lining of the digestive system, causing damage and inflammation. Soaking, sprouting, or fermenting nuts, seeds, grains, and legumes helps neutralize these inflammatory irritants.

Leaking in the gut can also affect the brain. Toxins from the guts that have leaked into the blood are one of the triggers of a "leaky brain." This occurs when substances that are normally kept out of the brain, such as heavy metals, bacteria, and environmental toxins, are able to breach the complex structure lining the capillaries of the brain known as the blood-brain barrier, leaving the brain susceptible to conditions that range from foggy thinking and poor short-term memory to more severe conditions like autism, depression, mental illness, seizures, chronic pain, and ADD/ADHD.

Keeping the Gut Healthy

Preservatives, GMOs, and the GAPS Diet

According to naturopathic physician Merrily Kuhn, RN, Ph.D, 80 percent of the food most Americans eat is genetically modified organisms (GMOs). The gut is not designed for GMOs, and they create bad bacteria in our guts. Most corn, sugar beets, and soy are genetically engineered. In addition to this, the words "natural flavor and natural spices" on product labels are extremely misleading and often refer to naturally derived sources that have been so processed they are as bad as or worse for us than the chemicals. Often missing from labels is monosodium glutamate (MSG). John Douillard notes, "As a flavor enhancer, MSG is required by the FDA to be listed in the ingredients. However, as a processing agent, which is very common in many food products, MSG does not require labeling."* The gut also can't handle products made with petroleum. Artificial flavors, colors, fragrances, and artificial perfumes are all chemicals that can be made from petroleum, including the commonly found synthetic compounds BHA, BHT, and TBHQ, which are used as antioxidants. Food additives, colorings, preservatives, refined sugars, MSG, and GMOs alter the gut microorganisms and can damage the intestinal wall.

---

*John Douillard, "Avoid Hidden MSG in the Health Food Aisle," John Douillard's LifeSpa, February 18, 2016, https://lifespa.com/sneaky-names-for-msg-check-your-labels.

Be mindful of what you are picking up off the shelf. The easiest choices are organic foods that come straight from the Earth, no processing. But if you are buying processed foods, read the labels. The bar code for organic foods is 94129. The bar code for GMO foods has five digits and begins with the number 8. There is an application for smartphones that will scan bar codes and check for good and bad ingredients. It will also tell you if it has preservatives and GMOs in it. See www.fooducate.com/about.

In addition to avoiding foods that will bring further damage to the gut, the GAPS program can help rebuild and restore healthy gut flora. *Gut and Psychology Syndrome: Natural Treatment for Autism, Dyspraxia, A.D.D., Dyslexia, A.D.H.D., Depression, Schizophrenia* was written by Natasha Campbell-McBride, MD, and inspired by the work of Dr. Sidney Valentine Haas, who treated damaged gut lining due to chronic inflammation in the digestive tract.

Probiotics

Probiotics are supplements or foods that contain lots of good bacteria. When you add probiotics to your diet, you help the good bacteria in your gut crowd out the bad bacteria.

One excellent source of probiotics is fermented foods. Among their beneficial bacteria are species that function as chelators; that is, they are able to bind with mercury, arsenic, and other heavy metals so they can be eliminated from the body through the stool. Kuhn recommended eating ¼ to ½ cup of fermented foods at least three or four times a week. She also suggested eating four different kinds of fermented foods regularly, to ensure a diverse probiotic supply. These fermented foods could include yogurt, kefir, sauerkraut, pickles, kimchee, and miso.

I myself have experienced great benefit from fermented tonics made from apple cider vinegar, garlic, onion, habanero pepper, ginger, horseradish, and turmeric, among other things. These ingredients contain powerful antibiotic, antiviral, and antifungal properties and boost blood and lymph circulation. Such tonics are very effective against colds, flu, and candida. When fermented, they become even more potent. My favorite version is the Earthie Mama Master Tonic, available at www.earthiemama.com.

True Anti-Aging

Today, with all the new information available about diet, our choice of how to feed ourselves can be confusing. It is vital to be discerning and to use science-based physiological information when making choices. No one diet is best for any one person, nor for any one person for their whole lifetime. Our nutritional requirements change throughout our lives. Needs vary from person to person, and we each have unique health challenges and lifestyle preferences.

Traditional cultures eat simple foods close to their natural forms. This is a good example to follow. Today's processed foods and sugars create tomorrow's problems. And remember this tip from nutritionist and energy worker Sybil Wander: "True anti-aging does not come from a miracle cream. It's an 'inside job.'"[30]

THE FIVE TIBETAN RITES

While living in Hawaii, I had the opportunity to do bodywork with a remarkable woman in her early nineties. One day before our session, she asked me to watch her do some exercises. In front of my very eyes, she proceeded to amaze me with cartwheels, handstands, headstands, and the splits in all three directions!

Then she showed me a series of abdominal strengthening exercises and yoga asanas. They looked like a combination of yoga and Pilates. These exercises were a part of her daily practice and were instrumental in her extraordinary vitality. She called these exercises the Five Tibetan Rites. She gave me a file with her handwritten notes, from which I obtained the following information.

As we've discussed, life-force energy flows in the body along the spine into seven primary energy centers or vortexes called chakras. Each chakra is associated with particular nerve plexuses, organs, and glands, including the body's seven major endocrine glands:

> **First chakra:** reproductive glands
> **Second chakra:** pancreas
> **Third chakra:** adrenal glands
> **Fourth chakra:** thymus gland
> **Fifth chakra:** thyroid gland
> **Sixth chakra:** pineal gland
> **Seventh chakra:** pituitary gland

In *Ancient Secret of the Fountain of Youth,* Peter Kelder writes,

In a healthy body, each of these spinning vortexes revolves at great speed, permitting vital life-force energy, also called prana or etheric energy, to flow upward through the endocrine system.

When all are revolving at high speed, and at the same rate of speed, the body is in perfect health. When one or more of them slows down, aging and physical deterioration set in. These spinning vortexes extend outward from the flesh in a healthy individual, but in the old, weak, and sickly they hardly reach the surface. The quickest way to regain youth, health, and vitality is to start these energy centers spinning normally again. There are five simple exercises that will help accomplish that. Any one of them alone is helpful, but all five are required to get the best results.[31]

The Five Tibetan Rites stimulate the flow of life-force energy through the chakras, enlivening nerves, organs, and glands. They also help lengthen and tone major muscle groups. My Line is enlivened daily by these rites. It takes me less than fifteen minutes to do twenty-one repetitions of each.

For the first week, perform each rite with just three repetitions. Each week, add a single repetition until you are doing twenty-one repetitions of each rite per day. You'll achieve optimal results with twenty-one repetitions, so there's no need to do more. The important thing is to be consistent and to do them daily. It helps to choose a convenient time and location in your home. I like doing the rites in my living room immediately upon arising. It is said that you can skip one day a week, but not more than that.

Special considerations: In the case of recent appendectomy or hernia, be cautious when performing the second and fifth rites. If you are overweight, be cautious with the fifth rite.

꩜ Normalizing Breaths between the Rites

In between the rites, practice this quick exercise to "normalize" your breath.

Stand with your hands on your hips and your feet about 4 inches apart. In this position, take a long, full, deep breath, inhaling through your nose.

Exhale through your mouth with your lips pursed in an O. Bend forward as you exhale audibly, sliding your hands down the front of your thighs until you are leaning on your knees. In this bent-forward position, squeeze every bit of breath out of your trunk, pulling your abdomen in tightly.

Then pull in and up at the pelvic floor, as though you are doing a Kegel exercise. Suck your belly button in toward your spine, and tuck your chin toward your chest. This tightens the three "locks" of your body: the pelvic lock, the abdominal lock, and the chin lock.

While holding your breath out and your abdomen in, slowly return to a fully upright position, sliding your hands back up to your hips. Continue holding your breath out for several seconds. Then take in a long, slow, deep inhale, and relax.

Then take two full, deep breaths, inhaling through your nose and exhaling through your mouth with your lips pursed in an *O*. This is to be done two times in between each rite.

⚘ Rite One

The first rite is done for the express purpose of speeding up the vortexes. Children do it all the time when they are playing. This rite also helps improve your balance.

Stand erect with your arms outstretched, fingers together, palms horizontal to the floor and spin clockwise, from left to right. To begin, turn slowly, and make sure your feet are turning as you spin. You may feel dizzy as you first begin. As you gently practice all five rites, the dizziness will abate.

To lessen the dizziness, focus your vision on a single spot straight ahead of you. As you begin to turn, hold your vision on that point as long as you can, then turn your head very quickly to refocus on that point. "Spotting" on that reference point will lessen your disorientation and dizziness.

When I stop spinning, I like to stabilize by separating my legs in a slight straddle position and bending my knees. If you feel like sitting or lying down to recover from any dizziness, by all means do so.

Count your spins as you go, building up from three to a maximum of twenty-one.

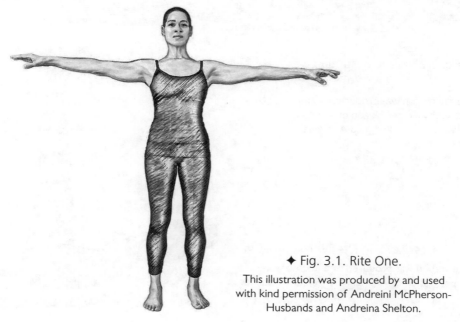

✦ Fig. 3.1. Rite One.

This illustration was produced by and used with kind permission of Andreini McPherson-Husbands and Andreina Shelton.

⚇ Rite Two

Lie flat on your back on a thick carpet or padded surface. Extend your legs straight out on the floor, with your ankles touching and your toes flexed upward. Extend your arms along the sides of your body, with your palms against the floor and your fingers close together.

Inhale through your nose, and as you do so, raise your legs, holding them straight, past a vertical position if possible. As you raise your legs, also raise your head off the floor, tucking your chin toward your chest. Do not let your knees bend. If you are unable to keep your knees perfectly straight, let them bend as needed.

Exhale, slowly lowering both your head and your straight legs back to the floor. Your lower back should not lift off the floor. Then allow all of your muscles to relax.

With each repetition of this rite, breathe in deeply as you lift your legs and head, and breathe out fully as you lower them. The more deeply you breathe, the better. Throughout the movement, consciously pull your belly down toward your back to strengthen your abdomen and to prevent disorganization of core-level muscles in the abdomen and pelvis.

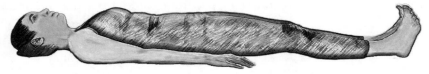

✦ Fig. 3.2. Rite Two: starting position.
This illustration was produced by and used with kind permission of Andreini McPherson-Husbands and Andreina Shelton.

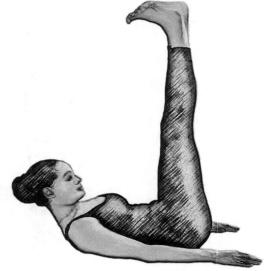

✦ Fig. 3.3. Rite Two: legs raised.
This illustration was produced by and used with kind permission of Andreini McPherson-Husbands and Andreina Shelton.

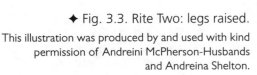

⚛ Rite Three

Kneel on the floor with your knees hip width apart and your feet flexed, so that your toes press into the floor. Place your hands against the sides of your legs. Lengthen along the front side of your spine through the top of your head, bending your head and neck forward and tucking your chin toward your chest.

Inhale through your nose, and as you do so, continue lengthening along the front of the spine as you bend your head and neck backward, gently arching your spine. Pull your belly button back to support your lumbar spine. Go only as far backward as you comfortably can. As you arch, press your arms and hands against the sides of your legs for support. Exhale through your mouth or nose as you return to your original position. Then repeat the rite.

Breathe in deeply as you arch backward. Breathe out as you return to an erect position. The lamas perform this rite with their eyes closed to help turn their attention inward.

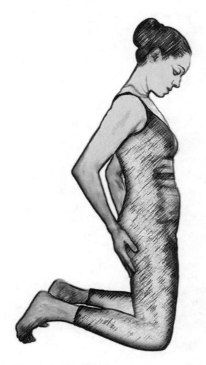

◆ Fig. 3.4. Rite Three: starting position.

This illustration was produced by and used with kind permission of Andreini McPherson-Husbands and Andreina Shelton.

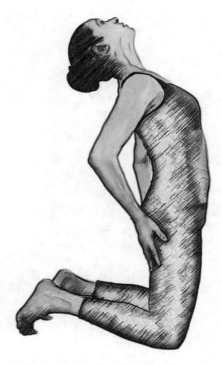

◆ Fig. 3.5. Rite Three: arched position.

This illustration was produced by and used with kind permission of Andreini McPherson-Husbands and Andreina Shelton.

⚘ Rite Four

Sit on the floor with your legs straight out in front of you and your feet about 12 inches apart. Holding the trunk of your body erect, place the palms of your hands on the floor alongside your hips. Tuck your chin forward toward your chest.

Inhale through your nose as you push down with your hands to lift your body while bending your knees and dropping your head back as far as it will go. Lift your torso as close to a table position as possible, parallel to the floor. Both your arms and lower legs will be straight up and down, perpendicular to the floor. As a beginner, you may find your table will sag. That's okay. It will improve over time.

While in the table position, tense every muscle in your body. Then relax and exhale, and as you do so, press down on your hands to lower your body back to its original sitting position, with your hips between your arms. Rest for a moment before you repeat the rite.

Breathe in deeply as you lift your body up. Hold in your breath as you tense your muscles. Breathe out completely as you lower your body. Then repeat.

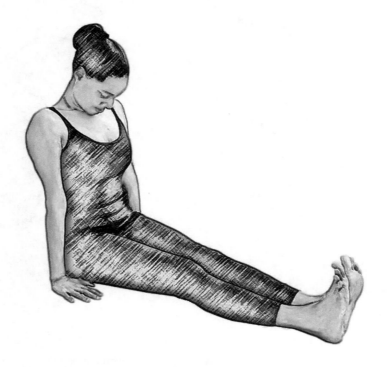

✦ Fig. 3.6. Rite Four: starting position.
This illustration was produced by and used with kind permission of
Andreini McPherson-Husbands and Andreina Shelton.

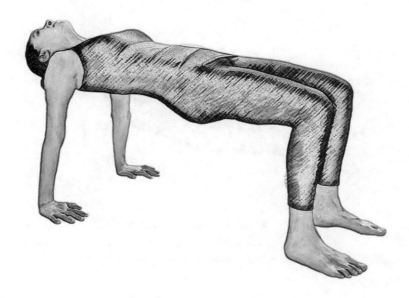

◆ Fig. 3.7. Rite Four: table position.

This illustration was produced by and used with kind permission of
Andreini McPherson-Husbands and Andreina Shelton.

Rite Five

Rite five is similar to a downward dog in yoga. Start in a push-up position, with
your arms perpendicular to the floor, your hands and feet shoulder width apart,
your legs straight, and your feet flexed, toes pushing into the floor. Traditionally,
this rite is done by arching the spine so that your abdomen almost touches the
floor with head held up and back as far as possible. However, I have learned that
to protect my lower back from curving excessively, I need to pull my abdomen in
and retain a flat back or plank position. This lessens the curve in my lower back at
the low point of this rite.

Then inhale through your nose, and as you do so, bend at the hips, pressing
down with your hands and feet to press your hips upward into an inverted V. At the
same time, drop your chin, tucking it toward your chest. Exhale through your nose
or mouth as you swing your body back down into its starting position.

Breathe in deeply as you raise your body. Breathe out fully as you lower it.
Repeat the rite. Tense your muscles for a moment, both at the raised point and at
the low point.

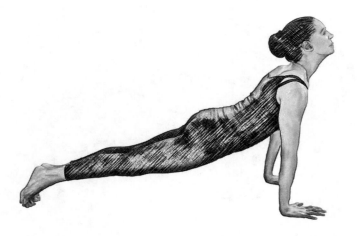

✦ Fig. 3.8. Rite Five: starting position (arched option).

This illustration was produced by and used with kind permission of
Andreini McPherson-Husbands and Andreina Shelton.

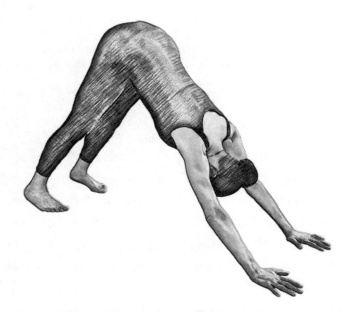

✦ Fig. 3.9. Rite Five: Inverted *V* position.

This illustration was produced by and used with kind permission of
Andreini McPherson-Husbands and Andreina Shelton.

◆ ◆ ◆

After completing all five rites, lie on your back and let your body rest. Notice
how you feel. I find these rites to be a great segue into my morning meditation
practice.

TENDING TO THE EMOTIONAL BODY

Detrimental Patterns
Affect the Body

Repetitive physical, behavioral, and emotional patterns can affect a person's physical, mental, and emotional bodies, which are all interrelated. If such patterns are out of balance, stress becomes embedded in the connective tissue as strain. *Strain is stress that has become internalized in the body.* A practitioner of Structural Integration can sense and feel some of those patterns in the body's tissues.

Examples of physical patterns that affect the body include sleeping more often on one side than the other, or habitually sitting with crossed legs. These types of physical patterns can put a twist into the body. So, too, can repetitive fearful thinking "tie a person up in knots"and lodge in the body as some form of strain or dis-ease.

In Structural Integration, we work with the physical body to help release stuck patterns of strain. Releasing these patterns can take some work, and I know from experience that a client does *not* want to put them back in. So it's important to understand sources of stress that may be creating problems in the body.

Often emotions can be a source of stress that creates patterns of strain. Let's take a closer look at how they can adversely affect the body.

Thoughts Affect the Nervous System

It is important to be mindful of the quality of one's thoughts. Thoughts have a powerful effect on the body due to the autonomic nervous system, which responds to a person's moods and is connected to internal organs.

The autonomic nervous system has two branches, called the sympathetic (fight or flight) and the parasympathetic (rest and repair). These two systems are designed to work in harmony with each other in order to balance the body. However, if the sympathetic nerves continually dominate, the body will begin to break down. If unchecked, degenerative processes and their symptoms can lead to full-blown health conditions that adversely affect the quality of one's life.*

---

*For more on this see www.holistichelp.net.

149

The sympathetic nerves run along each side of the spine from the first thoracic vertebra to the fourth lumbar vertebra. They respond to psychological or physiological stress by releasing the hormones adrenaline and cortisol. Adrenaline sharpens reflexes and prepares muscles for maximum exertion. Cortisol promotes the breakdown of the body's proteins to form glucose and acts as an anti-inflammatory and anti-allergenic. These hormones are designed for short-term use. In small doses, they work well. Problems arise when stress hormones are chronically released in the body.

The parasympathetic nerves, located at the brain stem and sacral area, help balance the effects of the sympathetic nerves. They activate the "rest and digest" mode of the body, increasing intestinal activity, slowing the heart rate, and lowering blood pressure after the "fight or flight" response has been activated.

The sympathetic and parasympathetic nerves are not under our direct control. Instead they respond to our emotions, which are affected by how we think. So how we think does affect our health.

Nervous Illness

A client of mine described a very stressful time in her life when she experienced panic attacks while attending law school. She searched bookshelves for an answer, and she cured herself of those disturbing episodes after reading and acting on the suggestions of Dr. Claire Weekes.

Dr. Weekes is known for her pioneering work in the study of nervous illness. The term *nervous illness* refers to people who suffer from anxiety and panic attacks, excessive fear, and disturbing physical nervous symptoms. In her book *Hope and Help for Your Nerves,* she noted: "A continuous state of fear, whatever the cause, gradually stimulates the adrenalin-releasing sympathetic nerves to produce a set pattern of disturbing sensations."[32]

According to Dr. Weekes, the disturbing physical symptoms may include "fatigue, churning of the stomach, indigestion, racing heart, banging heart, palpitations, 'missed' heartbeats, sweating hands, pins and needles in the hands, a choking feeling in the throat, an inability to take a deep breath, a tight feeling across the chest, sleeplessness, depression, nausea, occasional vomiting, diarrhea, and frequent urination."[33]

Consultation with a doctor can help determine whether the disturbing sensations originate from a physical problem in the body or from chronic stressful thought patterns that are creating physical symptoms of nervous illness—symptoms that, if unaddressed, could lead to more serious problems.

Discussing your condition with a wise counselor or friend is also important when you're dealing with nervous illness. Such a person can hold a bigger perspective for you during your time of recovery—a perspective that you may not be able to maintain on your own.

Pitfalls That Can Lead into Nervous Illness

Dr. Weekes described three main pitfalls that can lead into nervous illness: sensitization, bewilderment, and fear.

Sensitization

Sensitization is a state in which nerves react to stress in an exaggerated way, producing disturbing physical symptoms in the body very quickly. "The sensitized person puts himself in *a* cycle of fear-adrenalin-fear. His fear of the state he is in produces the adrenalin and other stress hormones, which continue to excite his nerves to produce the very symptoms he fears. The fear-adrenalin-fear cycle is also called an anxiety state."[34] "When a person is constantly sensitized, and afraid of the state he is in, we say he is nervously ill."[35]

Bewilderment

"Bewilderment acts by placing a sensitized person constantly under the strain of asking himself, 'What is wrong with me?' 'Why am I like this?' The more he struggles to be the person he was, the more stress he adds."[36]

Fear

Fear lies at the root of nervous illness. Fear sensitizes the body, causing fatigue and tension. It keeps a person in a state of anxiously wondering what will happen next. "So much nervous illness," said Dr. Weekes, "has no deep-seated cause and is no more than severe sensitization kept alive by bewilderment and fear."[37] "Symptoms can be intensified only by further fear and its resulting tension, never by facing and accepting."[38]

Dr. Weekes's Method of Recovery

"Thoughts that are keeping you ill can be changed," said Dr. Weekes. "We have no power to stop these reactions other than to change our mood." So how does a person do that? "Facing, accepting, floating and letting time pass will cure a person."[39]

Face the Fear

Facing means seeing a stressful thought for what it is—only a thought. We don't need to give so much attention to a thought and be controlled by it. Do not run away.

Accept

Regarding symptoms, Dr. Weekes suggests to "first relax and then examine and do not shrink from your symptoms. Go toward the symptoms and even describe them out loud to yourself. Understand your symptoms are the result of over-sensitization of adrenalin releasing nerves. . . . By true acceptance you break the fear-adrenalin-fear cycle. . . . Change your mood from apprehension to acceptance."[40] Fighting just brings on more symptoms.

Dr. Weekes stressed the importance of making sure one knows the difference between truly accepting and just putting up with it. "Acceptance means you are prepared to live and work with your symptoms while they are present without paying them too much respect. True acceptance means letting your stomach churn, letting your hands sweat and tremble, letting your heart thump without being too disconcerted by them."[41] "I stress acceptance," said Dr. Weekes, "because I have seen it cure while all else has failed."[42]

Floating

Allow the thoughts to float past and dissipate. When you think of floating, you relax and move or act more freely. Go on with whatever you were doing and do not pay them attention. There's no need to give them more energy and be drawn into them. Remember—they are just thoughts.

Letting Time Pass

"It will take time for your nerves to heal. If you are no longer afraid of your symptoms, and you are prepared to accept it and work with it, you will recover." It will not go away as soon as you stop fearing it. "It takes time for a body to establish acceptance as a mood and for this to eventually bring peace. That is why letting time pass is such an important part of the treatment."[43] "You recover by facing, accepting, floating and letting time pass."[44]

Thank you, Dr. Claire Weekes, for your brilliant work that has helped so many!

Taking Responsibility for Our Thoughts

I have found that I need to discriminate in the thoughts I think and *choose* what I give my attention to. Some thoughts may be worth thinking, and some I may want to dismiss and not entertain at all. In discerning the quality of a thought, I ask myself, "Is this a thought I want to continue thinking, or do I want to purify it and replace it with a more loving thought?"

The trick is to become the observer! That is, we must learn to see a thought from an objective perspective so that we can decide what we want to do with it. Perhaps the thought is one I would want to dismiss and stop it in its tracks before it can do any further harm! If a thought is abusive or fear based, I use the words "Out!" or "Stop!" to dismiss it immediately. In becoming the authority in this way, I can disintegrate the thought and release it from my brain.

Core Beliefs

Sometimes difficult thoughts arise that are related to core beliefs that no longer serve us. We have likely created them in response to past experiences that are no longer relevant in our lives, yet those accompanying feelings continue to have an effect on us. As core beliefs surface:

- ✦ Recognize the feeling that accompanies them
- ✦ Observe them so you can see what is necessary
- ✦ Become the authority and dismiss them and disintegrate them
- ✦ Bless and forgive yourself and know that the belief is all gone
- ✦ Repeat as necessary

Realizing that my beliefs were holding me back, I recently asked for my core beliefs to surface so I could clear them. Little did I know what a powerful practice that could be! As a core belief surfaces, it is often accompanied by intense emotion. So when I asked my core beliefs to emerge, emerge they did—and I began feeling awful! For weeks, I found myself suffering with old feelings that had come alive again. I wondered what had happened to me and why I was feeling that way.

Then I remembered my request for my core beliefs to emerge. The problem was, when they showed up, I became identified with them, instead of remaining the observer. When I became the observer, I was able to choose what to do with these beliefs and emotions. I was able to shift my focus and recognize the pattern I no longer wanted to perpetuate. It was a great learning experience! I just had to become the observer and allow them to release.

Responding to Thoughts with Compassion

In order to release certain patterns, we may need to attend and respond to some thoughts with compassion in order for them to release. A client of mine described this beautifully. Her teacher, Scott Wyman, a counselor in our area, calls this process "catch and release." Wyman suggests focusing on the difficult feeling or thought, giving it your attention and compassion, and slowly it will melt and release.

This is very similar to what a practitioner of Structural Integration does in the tissues of the body. I focus on a problematic area in the body with compassion and intend for it to release. Stuck tissue starts to move, and tension melts away. Then, energetically, that area is no longer isolated. The tissue can reintegrate into the rest of the body.

A Practice in Gratitude

For several years, I have participated in a gratitude practice with a group of dear women. We come together monthly to study and experience living in gratitude. This practice has been upgrading my life, and I am so grateful for it!

The books we have been studying are *Living in Gratitude: A Journey That Will Change Your Life,* by Angeles Arrien, and *The Magic,* by Rhonda Byrne. I cannot recommend these books enough! They have helped me replace negative thinking patterns with appreciation and joy. Through the inspiration of these books, my practice has become one of questing for the positive aspect and highest good even in the most difficult situations. I expect magnificent outcomes for things yet to happen in my life, and they occur!

"To *receive* you have to *give,*" says Byrne. "Gratitude is *giving* thanks.... *Thank you* must become the two words you deliberately say and feel more than any other words. They need to become your identity."[45]

"To experience the magic of gratitude in your life you have to practice it," says Byrne.[46] As we know, our feelings are powerful agents of change in our lives, whether for the positive or the negative. Our bodies are a composite of the physical, mental, and spiritual. We pattern these aspects of ourselves with how we think, feel, and do. Our thoughts, words, and actions *do* make a difference. Each moment can become a choice rather than a reaction.

Rick Hanson, Ph.D., neuropsychologist and author of *Hardwiring Happiness,* teaches positive psychology. He informs us that our brains are naturally drawn toward negative thinking. So intentionally reaffirming attitudes of gratitude strengthens our well-being.

"We can choose and choose again as the need arises," says Arrien, "to redirect our attention away from worries and resentment, shake ourselves loose from apathy and indifference, and focus our awareness—from moment to moment, hour by hour—upon tenderness and affection. We always have the opportunity and choice to express the love that flows between us and within our circle of influence, and extend it to all living peoples, creatures and plants."[47]

ESSENTIAL OILS

I love essential oils! Not only are they a powerful therapeutic tool, but they also bring a smile to my face and a lift to my heart as I smell their wonderful essence.

What Are Essential Oils?

Essential oils are the volatile liquids that are distilled from the roots, stems, bark, resin, rind, leaves, flowers, fruits, or seeds of plants. They have a strong electrical frequency that is much stronger than the measurable frequency of fresh produce and dry or fresh herbs. This strong electrical frequency makes them an excellent tool for physical, emotional, and spiritual healing.

Study of the biofrequency of humans and foods by Tainio Biologicals in Spokane, Washington, has shown that the human brain frequency is 72 to 90 megahertz (MHz). The human body registers 62 to 68 MHz during the day. Essential oils register anywhere between 52 and 320 MHz. Processed food has 0 MHz. Fresh produce measures up to 15 MHz. Fresh herbs are 20 to 27 MHz. Negative thoughts have been shown to lower the human frequency by 12 MHz, and positive thoughts raise the frequency by 10 MHz. Prayer and meditation raise the frequency by 15 MHz.[48]

In addition to their bioelectric potential, essential oils have dynamic chemical profiles, with hundreds of constituents. These chemical components can vary widely depending on the conditions of the plant growth, fertilizer, geographical region, climate, altitude, harvesting methods, and method of distillation.

The diversity of constituents enhances the effectiveness of the oils. A client of mine, who is a doctor of anesthesiology, described his successful use of essential oils to treat a MRSA infection that he had picked up from his work in the hospital. MRSA stands for "methicillin-resistant *Staphylococcus aureus.*" It's an infection caused by a strain of staph bacteria that have become resistant to powerful antibiotics. He said that the complexity of the chemical components in therapeutic-grade essential oils inhibits the MRSA bacteria from adapting to them.

Benefits of Pure Essential Oils

Because of the wide variances mentioned above, particularly in the methods of harvesting and distillation, it is important to know where and how your oils are sourced. It's important to use the purest oils possible to achieve the following benefits (and to avoid negative outcomes produced by poorly sourced oils).

- They increase oxygen and nutrients in the cells.
- They permeate every cell of the body within twenty minutes of ingestion or application.
- They are powerful antioxidants and free-radical scavengers.
- They detoxify the cells and blood.
- They have antibacterial, antifungal, antiparasitic, antiviral, antitumor, and anticancerous properties.
- They contain sesquiterpenes that can pass through the blood-brain barrier.
- When diffused, they provide air purification by removing toxins and metallic particles from the air while increasing oxygen levels.
- They promote physical, emotional, and spiritual well-being.
- They have a bioelectrical frequency that can quickly raise the frequency of the human body, helping to restore it to health.

I recommend the essential oils from Young Living (www.youngliving.com).

How Essential Oils Affect the Brain

Essential oils have profound effects not only physiologically but also psychologically. When inhaled, the oils go directly to the limbic system of the brain that stores and releases emotional trauma in the body. The limbic system also controls heart rate, blood pressure, breathing, memory, stress levels, and hormone balance.

The blood-brain barrier is the barrier membrane between the circulating blood and the brain that prevents certain damaging substances from reaching brain tissue and cerebrospinal fluid. . . . In June of 1994, it was documented by the

Medical University of Berlin, Germany and Vienna, Austria that sesquiterpenes have the ability to go beyond the blood-brain barrier. . . .

High levels of sesquiterpenes, found in the essential oils of frankincense and sandalwood, help increase the amount [of] oxygen in the limbic system of the brain, particularly around the pineal and pituitary glands. This leads to an increase in secretions of antibodies, endorphins, and neurotransmitters. . . .

Also present in the limbic system of the brain, is a gland called the amygdala. In 1989, it was discovered that the amygdala plays a major role in the storing and releasing of emotional trauma. The only way to stimulate this gland is with fragrance or the sense of smell. Therefore, with Aromatherapy and essential oils, we are now able to release emotional trauma.[49]

Being a bodyworker, I am aware that emotions get stuck in the organs, glands, tissues, and systems of the body. Carolyn L. Mein, chiropractor and author of *Releasing Emotional Patterns with Essential Oils,* states that emotions have frequencies just as each organ has a vibrational frequency. Emotions enter the body through the energy centers along the spine. From there, they move into the meridian system of the body through the connective tissues and settle into the DNA of the cells in an area with a corresponding frequency.[50]

Mein referenced Paul P. Pearsall, author of *The Heart's Code,* when she stated, "Transplant recipients report strange memories and desires which further substantiates that emotions are stored in the body and encoded in the DNA of cells."[51]

The high levels of sesquiterpenes found in the essential oils of frankincense and sandalwood, "help to increase the oxygen in the limbic system of the brain which in turn unlocks the DNA and allows emotional baggage to be released from cellular memory."[52]

Aromatic Use of Essential Oils

There are several ways to use the oils aromatically:

+ Pour two or three drops of the oil into the palm of your nondominant hand and use your other hand to rub the oil clockwise three times. This increases the electrical frequency of the oil. Then lift your palms to your nose, and inhale deeply.
+ Add a few drops of an oil to a bowl of water. Cover your head and the bowl with a towel and breathe deeply and slowly.
+ Use the oils in a diffuser. Look for one that does not use a heat source, as heat can alter the therapeutic benefit of the oil.

Topical Use of Essential Oils

Many essential oils are mild enough to be applied directly to the skin, while others need to be diluted in a carrier oil like extra-virgin olive oil or almond oil. Dilution of essential oils is *vital* for infants and small children. When dilution is required, a 1:10 ratio or greater is a good rule to follow. When applying an essential oil directly to your skin, use just 1 to 3 drops of the oil. Avoid touching the top of the bottle as that may contaminate the oil.

Essential oils can also be applied to contact points in the hands and feet in what is known as Vita Flex therapy, a form of reflexology. The term Vita Flex derives from the phrase "vitality through the reflexes," and it was coined by Stanley Burroughs, who is said to have brought this methodology to the United States from Tibet in the 1920s. Essential oils are applied to reflex points on a person's hands and feet by the fingertips of the practitioner, using a specific hand rotation. Because of the electrical nature of essential oils, vibrational healing energy then travels along meridians in the body to areas where it is needed.

Internal Use of Essential Oils

The internal use of essential oils is discouraged without the supervision of a qualified practitioner. Check the label of an essential oil for specifics, and never use an oil internally unless you're sure it's safe to do so.

Generally, essential oils are taken internally only in very small doses.

+ Several drops of food grade oil can be put into a vegetable capsule and swallowed with water.
+ One or two drops of the designated oil can be added to a glass of water, juice, yogurt, or plant-based milk.
+ One or two drops of oil can be added to a meal.

Raindrop Technique

In the Raindrop Technique developed by D. Gary Young, a sequence of pure grade essential oils is dropped directly onto the skin over the spine from 6 inches above the body and worked into the body with specific gentle strokes. The oils penetrate into the body's central nervous system, reaching cellular levels. Benefits include support of the immune system by killing off viruses that hibernate along the spinal column, reduction of spinal inflammation, straightening of spinal curvatures, rebalancing of the body at a structural/electrical level, and the release of emotional blockages from the past.

The height of a person is measured before and after a session. During a Raindrop session I received, my spine actually lengthened half an inch! In this technique, a session may take about an hour and will have beneficial effects for a week or more following the treatment.

By stimulating the central nervous system in this way, essential oils can be a valuable tool for balancing one's body, mind, emotions, and spirit!

MEDITATION AND THE QUANTUM FIELD

Neuroscience of the Mind-Body Connection

Meditation allows a person to focus his or her attention and quiet the mind. It is a powerful, personal tool to transform, energize, and organize mental and emotional bodies and, thereby, the physical body as well. Within the ever-changing depths of meditation, infinite layers of unfolding and letting go occur. Stress can be cleared from one's system, and a deep calm can nurture the spirit. It is also a way to reorient the compass of one's life and navigate through change.

Meditation is to my mental and emotional body what Structural Integration is to my physical body. Both allow for a more open and strong connection with my Line, my energetic channel to the source energies of the heavens and Earth.

The Quantum Field

Source energy is synonymous with the universal life-force energy of love and information, which doctor of chiropractic Joe Dispenza describes as the quantum field. His book, *You Are the Placebo,* combines information on current neuroscience and the mind-body connection.

This book has been a major influence in my life and has inspired me to return to a consistent meditation practice. That's where I experience big "me" time of energetic renewal. I look forward to my daily practices and consciously use meditation in both actively personal ways and receptive and universal ways.

During the actively personal part of my meditation, I engage thought, visualization, and emotion to consciously partner up with and direct energy of the quantum field. I ground, connect with heavenly and earthly energy, and clear stress out of my body. I partner up with the universal life-force energy and direct it to specific areas of my body for healing and for manifestation of my life choices.

During the receptive and universal phase, I relax in the present moment into the grace of the quantum field and allow it to bless me for my highest good. I observe and surrender to the infinite potential within that field. I drop into a deeper brain-wave state and become what Dispenza describes as "no thought, no body, and no time." The life-force energy in the quantum field helps my body to clear, organize, heal, renew, and optimize. This focused attention supports change in my physiology and progress on my life path.

In describing the quantum field, Dispenza writes:

> All particles are connected in an immaterial invisible field of information beyond space and time—and that field is made of consciousness (thought) and energy (frequency, the speed at which things vibrate). . . .
>
> Scientists are beginning to realize that a field of information exists that's responsible for myriad cellular functions existing beyond the boundaries of matter. It's this invisible field of consciousness that orchestrates all of the functions of the cells, tissues, organs, and systems of the body. It organizes matter to function in a harmonic, holistic way. . . .
>
> Call it what you will, but this is the universal intelligence that's giving you life right now. That intelligence loves you so much that it loves you into life. This invisible field of intelligence exists beyond space and time, and it's where all things material come from. Because it exists in all places and at all times, and it's both within you and all around you, this intelligence must be both personal and universal. So there's a subjective, free will consciousness called "you," and there's an objective consciousness that's responsible for all life.[53]

The human body is designed to be receptive to electromagnetic energy. It influences our cellular biology and genetic regulation. Science has determined that "the receptor sites on the outside of the body's cells happen to be a hundred times more sensitive to energy and frequency than they are to the physical chemical signals like neuropeptides, that we know gain access to our cells' DNA."[54]

Dispenza describes scientific research that states, "Specific frequencies of electromagnetic energy can influence the behavior of DNA, RNA, and protein synthesis; alter protein shape and function; control gene regulation and expression; stimulate nerve-cell growth; and influence cell division and cell differentiation, as well as instruct specific cells to organize into tissues and organs. All of these cellular activities influenced by energy are part of the expression of life."[55] What this means is that science now recognizes that energetic frequencies are the blueprint for life!

Our Interface
with the Quantum Field

How does the body regulate those expressions of life automatically? Through the autonomic nervous system, which Dispenza equates with the subconscious. The autonomic nervous system is our connection with the universal intelligence of life-force energy. It is within the autonomic nervous system that the automatic regulatory systems of the body function, such as heart rate, temperature, digestion, and hormone production. And how do we consciously gain access to effect change within the automatic operating system of the autonomic nervous system? Through emotion, Dispenza declares!

Emotions trigger the upregulation or downregulation—that is, the turning on or off—of genes. This is where epigenetics comes in. Our environment has significant impact on the expression of our genes. Genes create the proteins and chemicals that either build the body up or break the body down. Positive thoughts and emotions can trigger the upregulating of genes that are life enhancing. Negative emotions can activate genes that have a destructive influence on the body. It is literally mind over matter. Emotions help epigenetic changes happen faster. *in either direction.* Current neuroscience is validating the significance of this mind-body connection.[56]

How do I apply this in my meditation? I'll use the example of improving my eyesight. While in a deep, conscious part of my meditation, I will actively visualize both of my eyes having clear, full vision, and I'll feel what that would be like in my body. I'll add to that sense of feeling and visualization the strong emotion of gratitude, as though it has already taken place. The body then registers the healing from my mind and responds to it with the activation of genes that create the proteins and chemicals to express that.

"By bringing up the emotion of gratitude, *before* the actual event," says Dispenza, "your body (as the unconscious mind) will begin to believe that the future event has indeed already happened—or is happening to you in the present moment. Gratitude, therefore, is the ultimate state of receivership."[57]

According to Dispenza, when you focus strongly on an intention, your brain won't know the difference between reality and an inner thought that you desire to make more real. As the body begins to experience that focused intention in the present moment, it creates new genes to support it.

"If you continue to mentally practice enough times," says Dispenza, "your brain will begin to physically change—installing new neurological circuitry to begin to think from that new level of mind—to look as if the experience has already happened. You'll be producing the epigenetic variations that lead to real structural and functional changes in the body by thought alone. Then your brain and body will no longer be living in the same past; they'll be living in the new future that you created in your mind."[58]

Coherency and the Body as Particle and Wave

On an atomic level, the body is comprised of particles and waves. According to Dispenza, the particles are the material aspect of ourselves. The waves are the energetic aspect of our being.[59] During meditation, when we pay attention to the world within us, there is coherency, or order, created within the energetic aspect of our being. Atoms and molecules begin to vibrate faster. Different parts of the brain begin to organize and synchronize. The cells are able to communicate with one another as more energy becomes available. This heightened energetic state then informs the physical; it creates the blueprint that our bodies pattern after. The higher and more coherent our frequency is, the greater our health.

"So according to the quantum model of reality," says Dispenza, "we could say that all disease is a lowering of frequency. Think about stress hormones. When your nervous system is under the control of fight or flight mode, the chemicals of survival cause you to be more matter and less energy. . . . That means there is less consciousness, energy, and information available for atoms, molecules and chemicals to share. . . . This creates incoherence among the body's atoms and molecules, which causes a weakened signal of communication such that the body begins to break down."[60]

Meditation and
Brain-Wave States

It is within deep, conscious states of meditation that we can change patterns of mental and emotional strain in the brain that are affecting our bodies. How do we enter a state of meditation like that? By dropping from the conscious analytical mind of our outer world into a slower brain-wave state where we can access the subconscious mind of our inner world.

Brain-wave states can be measured through their frequency. The conscious analytical everyday waking state of the beta brain wave has a fast frequency. It processes sensory information and is not used for meditation. The next slower brain wave is alpha. This is the daydreaming brain-wave state. The inner world becomes more real as the frontal lobe is activated, which lowers the volume on sensory input and processing of time and space. Below the alpha brain wave is the deeper theta state. This is the slower brain-wave state that is best for meditation. It is here that people experience "the mind awake, the body asleep." It is also the brain-wave state where the mind is most suggestible.[61]

"Suggestibility," says Dispenza, "combines three elements: acceptance, belief, and surrender. The more we accept, believe, and surrender to whatever we're doing to change our internal state, the better the results we can create."[62]

Faith and grace are part of the meditation experience. I equate suggestibility with faith. We have to be able to let go of analytical judgments to be open to the possibility of change in the meditation experience. Grace is what happens in the quantum field. It is the infinite potential of that field to bless us.

Meditation
Requires Energy and Focus

Meditation creates a relationship with our own spiritual self. And like any relationship, it requires us to be present for it. I find that my best meditation sessions occur when I show up with energy and focus, so I prepare for meditation. Being a morning person—early to bed and early to rise—allows me to arrive fresh for my morning practice.

Dysfunctional patterns within the physical and energetic bodies may shift as a result of your meditation practice. This change can be uncomfortable and unfamiliar. If so, focus on observing what is going on with equanimity. Persevere as that stress clears. You may be dealing with not only your own stress, but what you have genetically and energetically inherited through your family line—the so-called "sins of the fathers." Know that even the physical genes we carry from our ancestors have the potential to change instantly through consciously present awareness in meditation. Through the depth and sincerity of your practice, the creation of your new coherent organized self will emerge.

IASI-Recognized Structural Integration Training Programs

Please be aware of the difference between the levels of training of a therapist who has taken a two-week workshop on Structural Integration and one who has completed a thorough, quality training that is recognized and compliant with the educational standards set by the International Association of Structural Integrators (IASI). IASI is the professional membership organization for Structural Integration that promotes the highest professional standards for Structural Integration. To find Structural Integration programs that are IASI recognized and currently compliant with its educational standards, visit the IASI website, www.theiasi.net.

Each of the IASI-recognized schools has developed out of Dr. Rolf's work and provides thorough certification programs and continuing education for Structural Integrators. They have similar and yet unique focuses of attention. Some of the earliest schools of Dr. Rolf's work include the following:

Guild for Structural Integration
150 S 600 E, Suite 1A, Salt Lake City, UT 84102
(801) 696-1169
www.rolfguild.org

In 1989, a small group of people formed the Guild for Structural Integration, an organization dedicated to preserving the original teachings of Dr. Ida P. Rolf. The Guild website states, "Association with the Guild implies not only a commitment to professional excellence in the performance of Dr. Rolf's standard ten-session series of Structural Integration, it also indicates a resolution to explore a path of personal growth which includes the transcendental vertical line."

Its mission statement says, "The vertical line is our fundamental concept. The physical and psychological embodiment of the vertical line is a way of BEING in the physical world. It forms a basis for personal growth and integrity."

Hellerwork Structural Integration International

Hellerwork International, 300 Avenida Adobe, San Clemente, CA 92672

(714) 873-6131

admin@hellerwork.com

http://hellerwork.com

Admissions Committee, ATT: Joseph Hunton

906 N 78th St, Seattle, WA 98103

Hellerwork Structural Integration was created by Joseph Heller. Heller became a Rolfer in 1972 and the first president of the Rolf Institute in 1975. He continued to study with Dr. Rolf through 1978, when he left the Rolf Institute to found Hellerwork Structural Integration.

Hellerwork Structural Integration addresses the psycho-emotional aspect of a person. Its added components of somatic psychology, movement education, and active therapeutic dialogue distinguish it from other forms of Structural Integration.

The Hellerwork website states, "Hellerwork is a system of bodywork that combines structural alignment, body movement education, and verbal dialogue. It is designed to realign the body's structure for overall health, improvement of posture, and reduction of physical and mental stress."

Hellerwork International is the international organization for all Hellerwork practitioners. Its mission is to "nurture the growth and integrity of Hellerwork in the world."

Rolf Institute of Structural Integration

5055 Chaparral Court, Suite 103, Boulder, CO 80301

(303) 449-5903

www.rolf.org

The Rolf Institute of Structural Integration was founded in 1971. It is head-quartered in Boulder, Colorado, and has international offices in Europe, Brazil,

Canada, and Japan. The vision of the Rolf Institute of Structural Integration is to provide "a quality training program in Rolfing Structural Integration, certifying Rolfers and providing them with continuing education, promoting research and educating the public about the value of Rolfing SI." The institute also partners with universities such as Harvard Medical School, UCLA, Stanford School of Medicine, and University of Sao Paulo in conducting research on Structural Integration.

Notes

FOREWORD

1. Goldthwait, "The Relation of Posture to Human Efficiency" and "The Conservation of Human Energy."
2. Hellebrandt and Franseen, "Physiological Study"; and Strait, Inman, and Ralston, "Sample Illustrations of Physical Principles."
3. Goldthwait, Brown, Swaim, and Kuhns, *Body Mechanics*.

PREFACE

1. Sise, *Rolfing Experience,* 229.
2. Feitis, *Ida Rolf Talks,* 14.
3. Feitis, *Ida Rolf Talks,* 88.

PART I. AN INTRODUCTION TO STRUCTURAL INTEGRATION

1. Feitis, *Ida Rolf Talks,* 31.
2. Rolf, *Rolfing,* 65.
3. Rolf, *Rolfing: Gravity Is the Therapist,* VHS.
4. Don Johnson, "Verticality and Enlightenment," 4.
5. Don Johnson, "Verticality and Enlightenment," 5.
6. Feitis, *Ida Rolf Talks,* 10.
7. Feitis, *Ida Rolf Talks,* 111.
8. Feitis, *Ida Rolf Talks,* 113.
9. Feitis, *Ida Rolf Talks,* 27, 31.
10. Sise, *Rolfing Experience,* 264.
11. Feitis, *Ida Rolf Talks,* 86.
12. Rolf, *Rolfing: Gravity Is the Therapist,* VHS.
13. Stone, *Polarity Therapy,* Chart no. 3, 10.
14. Feitis, *Ida Rolf Talks,* 206.
15. Oschman, *Energy Medicine,* 141.
16. Oschman, *Energy Medicine,* 73–74.
17. Oschman, *Energy Medicine,* 72.
18. Hunt, *Infinite Mind,* 19.

19. Oschman, *Energy Medicine,* 3.
20. Karl Maret, in Oschman, *Energy Medicine,* ix.
21. Oschman, *Energy Medicine,* 6.
22. Hunt, *Infinite Mind,* 88.
23. Albert Einstein quoted in Capek, *Philosophical Impact,* 319.
24. Hunt, *Infinite Mind,* 20.
25. Hunt, *Infinite Mind,* 48, 51.
26. Hunt, *Infinite Mind,* 49.
27. Hunt, *Infinite Mind,* 33.
28. Oschman, *Energy Medicine,* 61–62.
29. Oschman, *Energy Medicine,* 61–62.
30. Hunt, *Infinite Mind,* 12.
31. Hunt, *Infinite Mind,* 33.
32. Ober, Sinatra, and Zucker, *Earthing,* 44.
33. Oschman, in the foreword to Ober, Sinatra, and Zucker, *Earthing,* xii.
34. Oschman, in the foreword to Ober, Sinatra, and Zucker, *Earthing,* xii.
35. Ober, Sinatra, and Zucker, *Earthing,* 12.
36. Benias et al., "Structure and Distribution," https://www.nature.com/articles/s41598-018-23062-6.
37. Gibbens, "New Human 'Organ,'" https://news.nationalgeographic.com/2018/03/interstitium-fluid-cells-organ-found-cancer-spd.
38. Myers, "Understanding Fascia," 69.
39. Myers, "Understanding Fascia," 69.
40. Osborn, "Finding Fascia," 53.
41. Guimberteau, "The Living Fascia," 57.
42. "Biography," Dr. Jean-Claude Guimberteau, M.D., http://www.guimberteau-jc-md.com/en/biographie.php, "Basic Ideas."
43. "Biography," Dr. Jean-Claude Guimberteau, M.D., http://www.guimberteau-jc-md.com/en/biographie.php, "Basic Ideas."
44. "Biography," Dr. Jean-Claude Guimberteau, M.D., http://www.guimberteau-jc-md.com/en/biographie.php, "Basic Ideas."
45. Oschman, *Energy Medicine,* 74.
46. Oschman, *Energy Medicine,* 31.
47. Oschman, *Energy Medicine,* 99.
48. Oschman, *Energy Medicine,* 30.
49. Oschman, *Energy Medicine,* 57.
50. Oschman, *Energy Medicine,* 87.
51. Oschman, *Energy Medicine,* 87.
52. Feitis, *Ida Rolf Talks,* 124.
53. Feitis, *Ida Rolf Talks,* 124, 196.
54. Schleip and Muller, "Training Principles," 3.
55. Rolf, *Rolfing,* 171–72.

56. Quoted on a promotional flier created by Betsy Sise for the Guild for Structural Integration.

PART II. THE RECIPE SESSIONS

1. Feitis, *Ida Rolf Talks,* 181.
2. Heller and Hanson, *Client's Handbook,* 10.
3. Feitis, *Ida Rolf Talks,* 129.
4. Heller and Hanson, *Client's Handbook,* 12.
5. Rolf, *Rolfing,* 45.
6. Oschman, in the foreword to Ober, Sinatra, and Zucker, *Earthing,* xii.
7. Ober, Sinatra, and Zucker, *Earthing,* 66–67.
8. Rossi, "Walking."
9. Ober, Sinatra, and Zucker, *Earthing,* 4.
10. Ober, Sinatra, and Zucker, *Earthing,* 19.
11. Rossi, "Walking."
12. Ober, Sinatra, and Zucker, *Earthing,* 20.
13. Ober, Sinatra, and Zucker, *Earthing,* 19.
14. Heller and Hanson, *Client's Handbook,* 12.
15. Heller and Hanson, *Client's Handbook,* 14.
16. From class notes from a Postural Dynamics class that Dr. Rolf taught in Los Angeles in 1956. *Postural Dynamics* was the early name for Dr. Rolf's work.
17. Heller and Hanson, *Client's Handbook,* 15.
18. Heller and Hanson, *Client's Handbook.*
19. Heller and Hanson, *Client's Handbook,* 16.
20. Quoted by Emmet Hutchins during the author's auditing class at the Guild for Structural Integration in Boulder, Colorado, in July of 1991.
21. Sise, *Rolfing Experience,* 264.
22. Rolf, *Rolfing: Gravity Is the Therapist,* VHS.
23. Heller and Hanson, *Client's Handbook,* 18.
24. Rolf, *Rolfing,* 112.
25. Rolf, *Rolfing,* 113.
26. Heller and Hanson, *Client's Handbook,* 19.
27. Heller and Hanson, *Client's Handbook,* 19.
28. Heller and Hanson, *Client's Handbook,* 20.
29. Rolf, *Rolfing,* 125.
30. Feitis and Schultz, "A Rolfian Review of Anatomy," 17.
31. From notes from a six-day continuing education workshop in Kauai, Hawaii, in February of 2012 with Emmett Hutchins.
32. Heller and Hanson, *Client's Handbook,* 21.
33. Heller and Hanson, *Client's Handbook,* 22.
34. Rolf, *Rolfing,* 231.
35. Heller and Hanson, *Client's Handbook,* 22.
36. Heller and Hanson, *Client's Handbook,* 20–21.

37. Heller and Hanson, *Client's Handbook,* 24.
38. Rolf, *Rolfing,* 189.
39. Heller and Hanson, *Client's Handbook,* 24–25.
40. Heller and Hanson, *Client's Handbook,* 25.
41. Heller and Hanson, *Client's Handbook,* 26.
42. Sise, *Rolfing Experience,* 100.
43. Sise, *Rolfing Experience,* 98.
44. Heller and Hanson, *Client's Handbook,* 27.
45. Heller and Hanson, *Client's Handbook,* 25.
46. Heller and Hanson, *Client's Handbook,* 27.
47. Heller and Hanson, *Client's Handbook,* 28.
48. Rolf, *Rolfing,* 249.
49. Rolf, *Rolfing,* 289.
50. Heller and Hanson, *Client's Handbook,* 29.

PART III. SUPPORT TOOLS

1. Swiss Bionic Solutions USA, "Earth's Magnetic Field," iMRS.com, http://www.imrs.com/en/earth-s-magnetic-field.html.
2. Hunt, *Infinite Mind,* 30–32.
3. Nichols, "16 Science-Backed Health Benefits," https://www.well-beingsecrets.com/health-benefits-of-far-infrared-rays.
4. Nichols, "16 Science-Backed Health Benefits," https://www.well-beingsecrets.com/health-benefits-of-far-infrared-rays.
5. Sears, Kerr, and Bray, "Arsenic, Cadmium, Lead, and Mercury."
6. Beever, "Far-Infrared Saunas."
7. Ishibashi et al. "Effects Inhibiting Proliferation of Cancer Cells."
8. Nichols, "16 Science-Backed Health Benefits," https://www.well-beingsecrets.com/health-benefits-of-far-infrared-rays.
9. Young and Young, *The pH Miracle,* 77.
10. Young and Young, *The pH Miracle,* 91.
11. Young and Young, *The pH Miracle,* 11–12.
12. Young and Young, *The pH Miracle,* 5.
13. Young and Young, *The pH Miracle,* 31.
14. Young and Young, *The pH Miracle,* 31.
15. Young and Young, *The pH Miracle,* 40.
16. Sircus, *Magnesium for Life,* 12.
17. Young and Young, *The pH Miracle,* 13–14.
18. As presented by Kuhn in a seminar for the Institute for Brain Potential in Chico, California, "Understanding the Gut Brain: Stress, Appetite, Digestion and Mood."
19. Young and Young, *The pH Miracle,* 82.
20. Young and Young, *The pH Miracle,* 123.
21. Young and Young, *The pH Miracle,* 125.

22. Young and Young, *The pH Miracle,* 67.

23. Young and Young, *The pH Miracle,* 66.

24. Young and Young, *The pH Miracle,* 82.

25. Young and Young, *The pH Miracle,* 82.

26. Young and Young, *The pH Miracle,* 27.

27. Young and Young, *The pH Miracle,* 15.

28. Deborah Johnson, *Home Test pH Kit,* 14.

29. Deborah Johnson, *Home Test pH Kit,* 15.

30. Deborah Johnson, *Home Test pH Kit,* 5.

31. Kelder, *Ancient Secret,* 11.

32. Weekes, *Hope and Help,* 8.

33. Weekes, *Hope and Help,* 10.

34. Weekes, *Peace from Nervous,* 6.

35. Weekes, *Hope and Help,* 13.

36. Weekes, *Peace from Nervous,* 6.

37. Weekes, *Peace from Nervous,* 7.

38. Weekes, *Hope and Help,* 34.

39. Weekes, *Hope and Help,* 2, 5.

40. Weekes, *Hope and Help,* 26, 27, 29.

41. Weekes, *Hope and Help,* 33.

42. Weekes, *Peace from Nervous,* 56.

43. Weekes, *Hope and Help* 27, 29.

44. Weekes, *Hope and Help,* 72.

45. Byrne, *Magic,* 17–18.

46. Byrne, *Magic,* 10.

47. Arrien, *Living in Gratitude,* 44.

48. Higley and Higley, *Reference Guide,* 4.

49. Higley and Higley, *Reference Guide,* 5.

50. Mein, *Releasing Emotional Patterns,* 6.

51. Quoted in Mein, *Releasing Emotional Patterns,* 5.

52. Mein, *Releasing Emotional Patterns,* 6.

53. Dispenza, *You Are the Placebo,* 188, 191, 197.

54. McClare, "Resonance," referenced in Dispenza, *You Are the Placebo,* 179.

55. Dispenza, *You Are the Placebo,* 179–80.

56. Dispenza, *You Are the Placebo,* 112.

57. Dispenza, *You Are the Placebo,* 135.

58. Dispenza, *You Are the Placebo,* 105.

59. Dispenza, *You Are the Placebo,* 186.

60. Dispenza, *You Are the Placebo,* 192–93.

61. Dispenza, *You Are the Placebo,* 152–54.

62. Dispenza, *You Are the Placebo,* 130.

Bibliography

Arrien, Angeles. *Living in Gratitude: A Journey That Will Change Your Life.* Boulder, Colo.: Sounds True, Inc., 2011.

Beever, R. "Far-Infrared Saunas for Treatment of Cardiovascular Risk Factors: Summary of Published Evidence." *Canadian Family Physician* 55, no. 7 (July 2009): 691–96.

Benias, Petros C., Rebecca G. Wells, Bridget Sackey-Aboagye et al. "Structure and Distribution of an Unrecognized Interstitium in Human Tissues." *Scientific Reports* 8 (March 27, 2018), https://www.nature.com/articles/s41598-018-23062-6.

Byrne, Rhonda. *The Magic.* New York: Atria Books, 2012.

Capek, Milic. *The Philosophical Impact of Contemporary Physics.* New York: Van Nostrand Reinhold, 1961.

Dispenza, Joe. *You Are the Placebo: Making Your Mind Matter.* Carlsbad, Calif.: Hay House, 2014.

Elgin, Duane. *The Living Universe: Where Are We? Who Are We? Where Are We Going?* San Francisco: Berrett-Koehler, 2009.

Feitis, Rosemary, ed. *Ida Rolf Talks about Rolfing and Physical Reality.* New York: HarperCollins, 1979.

Feitis, Rosemary, and R. Louis Shultz. "A Rolfian Review of Anatomy." *Rolf Lines* 22, no. 1 (January 1994): 13–18.

Gibbens, Sarah. "New Human 'Organ' Was Hiding in Plain Sight." *National Geographic,* March 27, 2018, https://news.nationalgeographic.com/2018/03/interstitium-fluid-cells -organ-found-cancer-spd.

Goldthwait, J. E. "The Conservation of Human Energy: A Plea for a Broader Outlook in the Practice of Medicine." *Rocky Mountain Medical Journal* 19 (1911): 341–50.

———. "The Relation of Posture to Human Efficiency and the Influence of Poise upon the Support and Function of the Viscera." *Boston Medical and Surgical Journal* 161 (1909): 839–48.

Goldthwait, J. E., L. T. Brown, L. T. Swaim, and K. G. Kuhns. *Body Mechanics in the Study and Treatment of Disease.* Philadelphia: J. B. Lippincott, 1943.

Guimberteau, Jean-Claude. "The Living Fascia: Rethinking Our Assumptions." *Massage & Bodywork,* September/October 2016, 57.

Hellebrandt, F. A., and E. B. Franseen. "Physiological Study of the Vertical Stance of Man." *Physiological Review* 23 (1943): 220–55.

Heller, Joseph, and Jan Hanson. *The Client's Handbook: Hellerwork.* Body of Knowledge, Inc., and Hellerwork Practitioners Assn., 1990.

Higley, Connie, and Alan Higley. *Reference Guide for Essential Oils.* Olathe, Kans.: Abundant Health, 1998.

Hunt, Valerie V. *Infinite Mind: Science of the Human Vibrations of Consciousness.* Malibu, Calif.: Malibu Publishing Company, 1996.

Ishibashi, J., K. Yamashita, T. Ishikawa et al. "The Effects Inhibiting the Proliferation of Cancer Cells by Far-Infrared Radiation (FIR) Are Controlled by the Basal Expression Level of Heat Shock Protein (HSP) 70A." *Medical Oncology* 25, no. 2 (2008): 229–37.

Johnson, Deborah Page. *Home Test pH Kit.* Naperville, Ill.: NewPage Productions, 2012.

Johnson, Don Hanlon. *Bone, Breath, and Gesture: Practices of Embodiment,* vol 1. Berkeley, Calif.: North Atlantic Books, 1995.

Johnson, Don Hanlon. "Verticality and Enlightenment." *Somatics,* Fall/Winter 1993, 5.

Kelder, Peter. *Ancient Secret of the Fountain of Youth,* Book 1. Gig Harbor, Wash.: Harbor Press, Inc., 1985.

McClare, C. F. W. "Resonance in Bioenergetics." *Annals of the New York Academy of Sciences* 227 (1974).

Mein, Carolyn L. *Releasing Emotional Patterns with Essential Oils.* Rancho Santa Fe, Calif.: Vision Ware Press, 1998.

Myers, Thomas W. *Anatomy Trains: Myofascial Meridians for Manual & Movement Therapists.* Amsterdam: Elsevier Ltd., 2014.

——. "Understanding Fascia: The Radical Story of an Adaptive System." *Massage & Bodywork,* September/October 2016, 69.

Nichols, Helen. "16 Science-Backed Health Benefits of Far-Infrared Rays." Well-Being Secrets, https://www.well-beingsecrets.com/health-benefits-of-far-infrared-rays.

Ober, Clinton, Stephen T. Sinatra, and Martin Zucker. *Earthing: The Most Important Discovery Ever?* Laguna Beach, Calif.: Basic Health Publications, 2010.

Osborn, Karrie. "Finding Fascia." *Massage & Bodywork,* September/October 2016, 53.

Oschman, James. *Energy Medicine in Therapeutics and Human Performance.* Edinburgh: Butterworth Heinemann, Elsevier Limited, 2003.

——. *Energy Medicine: The Scientific Basis.* 2nd ed. Amsterdam: Elsevier, 2016.

Rolf, Ida P. *Rolfing: Reestablishing the Natural Alignment and Structural Integration of the Human Body for Vitality and Well-Being.* Rochester, Vt.: Healing Arts Press, 1989.

——. *Rolfing: The Integration of Human Structures.* Santa Monica, Calif.: Dennis-Landman, 1977.

Rossi, William A. "Walking on Touch-Deadened Feet." *Footwear News* 53, no. 50 (December 15, 1997): 20.

Schleip, Robert, and Divo Gitta Muller. "Training Principles for Fascial Connective Tissues: Scientific Foundation and Suggested Practical Applications." *Journal of Bodywork & Movement Therapies* 17, no. 1 (2013): 103–15.

Sears, M. E., K. J. Kerr, and R. I. Bray. "Arsenic, Cadium, Lead, and Mercury in Sweat: A Systemic Review." *Journal of Environmental Public Health,* no. 184745 (February 2012): Epub, doi: 10.1155/2012/184745.

Sircus, Mark. *Magnesium for Life.* 2006, http://www.spiritofhealthkc.com/wp/wp-content/uploads/2014/03/MAGNESIUM-Magnesium-for-Life.pdf.

Sise, Betsy. *The Rolfing Experience: Integration in the Gravity Field.* Prescott, Ariz.: Hohm Press, 2005.

Stone, Randolph. *Polarity Therapy: The Complete Collected Works on this Revolutionary Healing Art by the Originator of the System,* volume 2. Summertown, Tenn.: Book Publishing Company, 1987.

Strait, L. A., V. T. Inman, and H. J. Ralston. "Sample Illustrations of Physical Principles Selected from Physiology and Medicine." *American Journal of Physiology* 15 (1947): 375–82.

Weekes, Claire. *Hope and Help for Your Nerves.* New York: New American Library, 1969.

———. *Peace from Nervous Suffering.* New York: Hawthorn Books, 1972.

Young, Robert O., and Shelley Redford Young. *The pH Miracle: Balance Your Diet, Reclaim Your Health.* New York: Grand Central Life & Style, 2002.

Audiovisual Recordings

Gamble, Foster, and Kimberly Carter Gamble. *Thrive: What on Earth Will It Take?* DVD. Soquel, Calif.: Clear Compass Media, 2011, www.thrivemovement.com/the_movie.

Rolf, Ida. *Rolfing: Gravity Is the Therapist.* VHS. Boulder, Colo.: Rolf Institute of Structural Integration, 1976.

Index

Page numbers in *italics* indicate illustrations.

About the Author

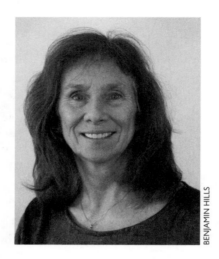

BENJAMIN HILLS

Jean Louise Green became a licensed massage therapist in the state of Hawaii in 1987. She received her certification as a practitioner of Structural Integration in the Dr. Ida Rolf Method with the Guild for Structural Integration in 1991. Green is a professional member of the International Association of Structural Integrators (IASI) and the Guild for Structural Integration.

From 2005 to 2018 Green was a California state-certified teacher of basic and advanced level deep tissue classes and senior staff member of the Chico Therapy Wellness Center, a massage school in Chico, California. Her knowledge of body structure and mechanics made her classes highly valuable for massage therapists working in the healing arts. Green maintains a vibrant Structural Integration practice where she lives and works in Chico, California.